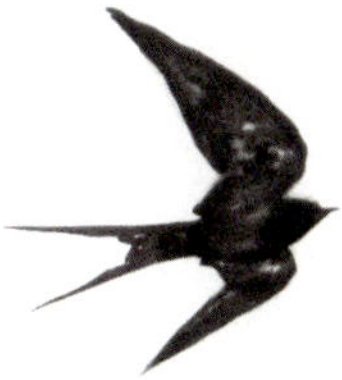

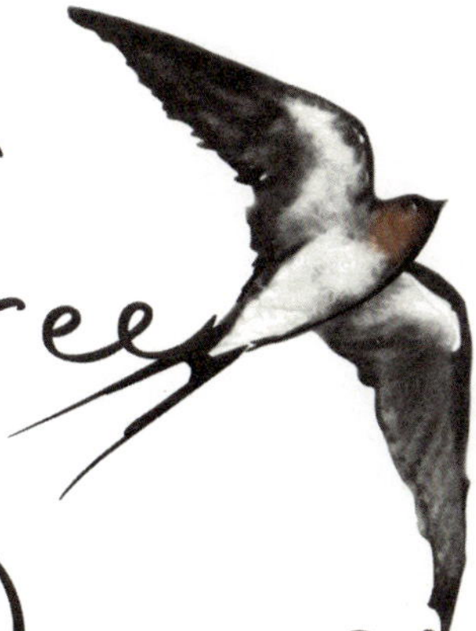

Free Dancing

RANDOM STORIES FROM AN ACCIDENTAL LIFE

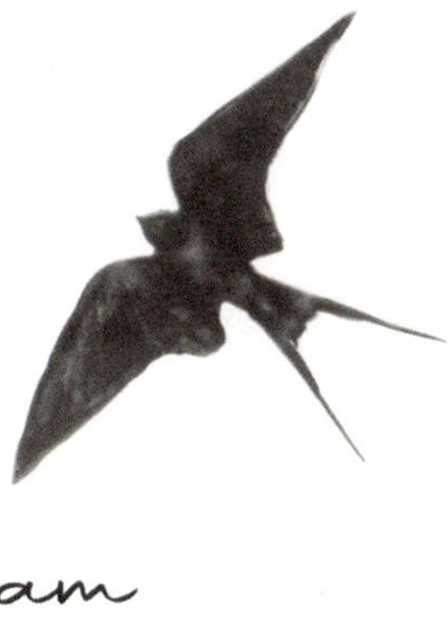

Ken Brigham

Free Dancing

Secant Publishing, LLC
P.O. Box 4059
Salisbury MD 21803
www.secantpublishing.com

ISBN 978-1-7359957-1-7 (hardcover)
ISBN 978-1-7359957-2-4 (ebook)

FREE DANCING

Random Stories from an Accidental Life

KEN BRIGHAM

Secant Publishing
SALISBURY, MARYLAND

To Arlene, Heather, and Josh

They taught me to love and be loved.

BOOKS BY THE AUTHOR:

Nonfiction:

Hard Bargain

With Michael M.E. Johns

Predictive Health

The Good Doctor

Fiction:

The Life and Deaths of Blanche Nero

Deadly Science

Deadly Arts

With Neil Shulman

Spotless

The Asolo Accords

Technical works edited

Respiratory Distress Syndromes

Endotoxin and the Lungs

Gene Therapy for Diseases of the Lungs

www.kenbrigham.com

"...that's what life is like, in the end. Not a novel.
A sliced loaf of short stories. But with different grains."

— Martin Amis, *Inside Story*

Swallows dance in the early spring evenings. The mature ones glide in formation as though driven by a common purpose, a communal intent, that gathers them into a clear pattern and heads the patterned group in a mutually agreed upon direction toward presumably a mutually agreed upon goal. At least it looks that way from our Southeast facing Atlanta balcony around nine o'clock on a particularly amiable moonlit night. Watching them is a dance lesson. Arthur Murray could learn something.

But the youngsters were the opening act, delighting in the liberation of flight with no worries about order. Free dancing, Arlene calls it. Each cavorting to their private music, darting hither and yon and somehow avoiding collisions, their innate sense of impending danger instructing them to nip deftly to port or starboard at the very last critical moment. Whew, that was close. Be careful, kids. There is a thrill to be had in taking chances, but risks don't always work out so well. You will learn that soon enough.

That's one way to live, free dancing. It carries some risk, but there is something to be said for it.

Contents

Discovery

Change

Opportunity

Non Finito

Answers

Questions

Why? Why Not?

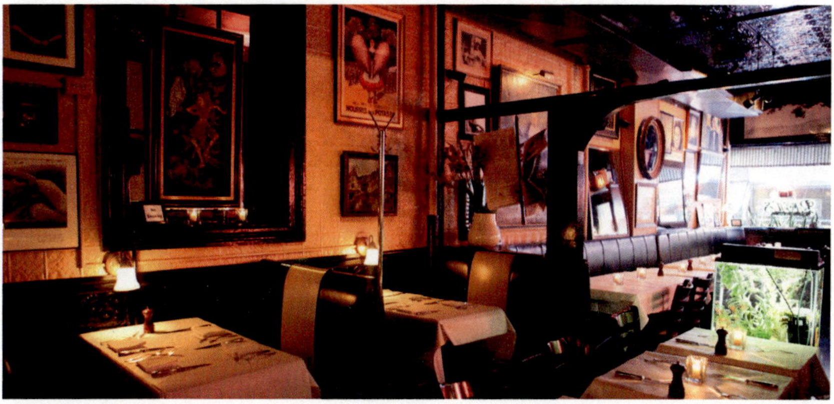

Courtesy of Raoul's

Raoul's

Accidents happen. They are integral to the human condition. I, for one, am living proof. Or at least I think so.

Were it not for an accident of social history and parental inclinations, I am quite sure that I would not exist. In 1939, the business of family planning was not so precise as in later generations. Thus, the fact of my birth in that year when my father was 50 and my mother 38, and having two siblings who had already lived a third or so of a generation, completely convinces me that I was not an intended consequence of normal conjugal activity. I think I just happened. An accident, but a happy one, for the most part ... maybe biology free dancing.

Why?

The seed for this book was planted at Raoul's, a pub-cum-restaurant in Greenwich Village—another accident of sorts. Heather (my daughter) and Josh (her husband) joined Arlene (my wife) and me in the city to celebrate Heather's birthday. During dinner the three of them drifted into a conversation about my life which they opined was something different than what its accidental beginning and largely unpromising early years might have portended. Since I now had time and had taken up writing as pretty much a full-time avocation, they figured that I should write my life story.

The seed was not quick to germinate. That's because, try as I might, I couldn't see my life as anything resembling a story—something with a beginning, middle, and end that segued easily into one another. I finally concluded that while I have had the enormous privilege of participating in a lot of interesting and enriching experiences, they do not sum up to a story. Rather than a story, my life was (and continues to be, I think) an olio of largely unconnected anecdotes. Just try to connect these dots—farm boy, pop star, doctor, scientist, biotech entrepreneur, world traveler, cancer survivor, medical administrator, author. If you succeed, your capacity for mental gymnastics is greater than mine. So, I am the enormously fortunate heir of numerous by and large wonderful but unconnected anecdotes, mostly accidents. I'm not surprised by that given my accidental origin. Maybe I inherited the great good fortune of being accident-prone.

What follows is a collection of some of those anecdotes as I remember them. With deference to the order of our cosmos, I arrange the nine sections sequentially as I remember time, but the individual stories are patched together in no particular order. It is irrational to imagine an integral pattern to free dancing and anyway orderly memory has pretty much splintered beyond recognition by the time one's age passes the four-score milestone.

So, these are just some things that I remember, how I remember them, and some thoughts about them that are as anecdotal as the stories. They are best read as individual essays. There are real people whom I admire and respect and the events are true to my no doubt imperfect memory of them; others may recall things differently. Like the man said, *memory is a work of the imagination*. That's perfectly fine with me. I mean, after all ...

Why not?

Being

The Angst of Cees

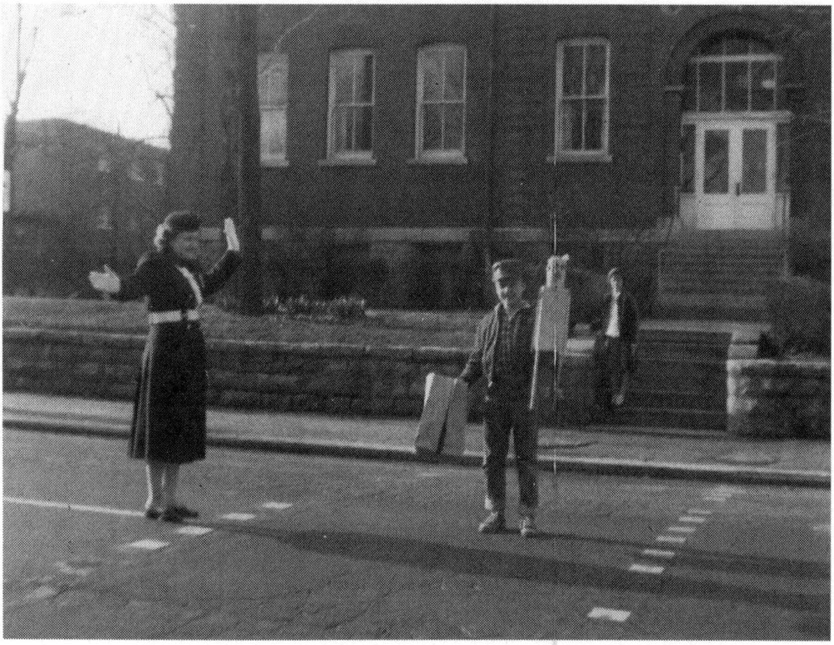

Nashville Public Library Metro Nashville Archives

Glenn Elementary School

The ages of five and six years, when one starts formal schooling, and cracks, ever-so-timid ones, begin to appear in the doors that promise to open up to the wider world, should be heady times for kids. New friends. New adventures. The exhilaration of learning new things. It didn't happen that way for me.

Mostly, I cried. If Miss Elizabeth Hendricks, the lanky olive-skinned schoolmarm (that seems on reflection an appropriate, if outmoded, title for her) with braided black hair encircling her head, who taught first and second grades, paid attention to me, I cried. If she ignored me, I also cried. There was pretty much nothing that could happen in that classroom at Nashville's Glenn Elementary School that I would respond to with anything other than tears.

And not just tears. We're talking gut-wrenching sobs. My severely limited repertoire of reactions to my newly imposed educational opportunity was, I am sure, a matter of utter frustration to the people in charge. Miss Hendricks probably shook her head and rolled her eyes heavenward when describing my behavior to her colleagues in the teachers' lounge.

And I was deathly afraid of being late. From the time I arose in the morning until I collected my book satchel and headed for another lachrymose day in the world of elementary education, I chanted a white rabbit-like mantra: *I'm gonna be late; I'm gonna be late*. In fact, I was always very early, arriving before the doors were unlocked and sitting patiently on the front steps until someone arrived and let me in. But no matter how sincere and repeated my mother's assurances that I was not going to be late, that the principal had complained that I was always there too early, her pleas were to no avail.

I was never late. In fact, I don't think I have ever been late for anything in my entire life. Habits (or perhaps neuroses) form early, I suppose.

There must be some profound lesson in the way Miss Hendricks (probably in consultation with colleagues) chose to approach my incessant crying problem. Hit him where it hurts, in his report card. I anxiously awaited that record of my performance at the end of each grading period. Mine was always filled with A's; my worth as a person was bound up in that. But I was never confident that the A's would be there until I had the hard evidence in hand. You can imagine the impact of a C glaring out from among the sea of A's. All A's except a C in conduct with a note explaining that the C was because I cried so much in class. Of course, that grade triggered a prolonged bout of uncontrollable weeping. Not, I am sure, the response that Ms. Hendricks sought. Despite that, she stuck with the conduct C accompanied by the explanatory note through several grading cycles, always with the same result. Her tactic was a miserable failure. It took her a while to learn that fear and insecurity are not so easily dealt with, although she surely racked up some chits in the Great Book of

Life for her persistence. Punishment is not a good way to approach problems that are beyond the control of the behaver. Beating a dead horse, no matter how nobly motivated, is rarely either satisfying or effective.

So, I was a hopelessly neurotic kid. How come? I had a stable home. I was not mistreated. We were poor, but we had plenty to eat and we were clothed and housed adequately. I remember much of that period of my life vividly, but I don't remember being unhappy most of the time. I do remember being afraid that I was living in a house of cards, that something of major proportion might go wrong and the whole thing would collapse. And, even worse, that it could be my fault. I'd better be very careful.

This was 1944, 1945. Maybe it had something to do with the war.

The Good War wasn't good for everybody. Young men disappeared from North Seventh Street where I lived and some of them never returned. Sometimes I would see my parents late of an evening sitting at the kitchen table counting out the ration stamps (sugar, gas), carefully detached from a little brown packet, and talking seriously in hushed tones, frowning. The words I heard broadcast from our black plastic Motorola tabletop radio were scary words: people killed on a scale that I couldn't comprehend; an evil dictator run amok in the world; the grinding crunch of battalions of boots marching who knew where, scrunch, scrunch, scrunch; American citizens forced away from their homes to camps somewhere out West.

And eventually, the bomb. Destruction on a cosmic scale. Good God, what if that was my fault, somehow related to my being late to school or getting a C on my report card? I didn't see how that could be, but then at ages five and six, I didn't understand much about why things happened like they did. I was sure that adults were not telling me a lot about how the world worked, but I wasn't about to ask. I was afraid of what the answers might be.

The Good War hit home. In 1944, my half brother-in-law (his wife was my father's daughter from his first marriage; her mother died in the 1918 flu pandemic), drafted into the army and sent with his wife and two children to South Carolina, killed his wife and himself. I never heard the circumstances discussed; perhaps I was protected. Whatever the story was, it would be hard not to conclude that the two young people were casualties of what came to be known as The Good War. Their son went to live with his father's parents and their daughter (technically my half-niece, just a year older than I was) came to live with us and has remained essentially my sister to this day. She is a good woman who has made for herself, her family, and others a good life. She has done so in spite of suffering potentially devastating collateral damage from the war. As a child, she was more at peace than I was. That baffles me. Some sociopsychologist must have done a study of the kids who were just entering the wider world around that time. Maybe we are a distinct group—*children of The Good War.*

Had my family been more affluent and had the times been different, I would probably have spent a substantial number of hours with a therapist. As I remember what kind of a child I was, I suspect that things would not have gone well in such a situation. I would either have consumed each session with prolonged periods of uncontrollable weeping or I would have tried desperately (and transparently to a good therapist) to say whatever I thought would please her, revealing as little as possible about the reality of myself; not much substance for a therapist to work with. Would I have been a happier, more well-adjusted, better functioning child? Maybe. But I doubt if, in the long run, my life would have turned out any better. I'm not sure that therapists put a lot of faith in free dancing.

Living Land to Mouth

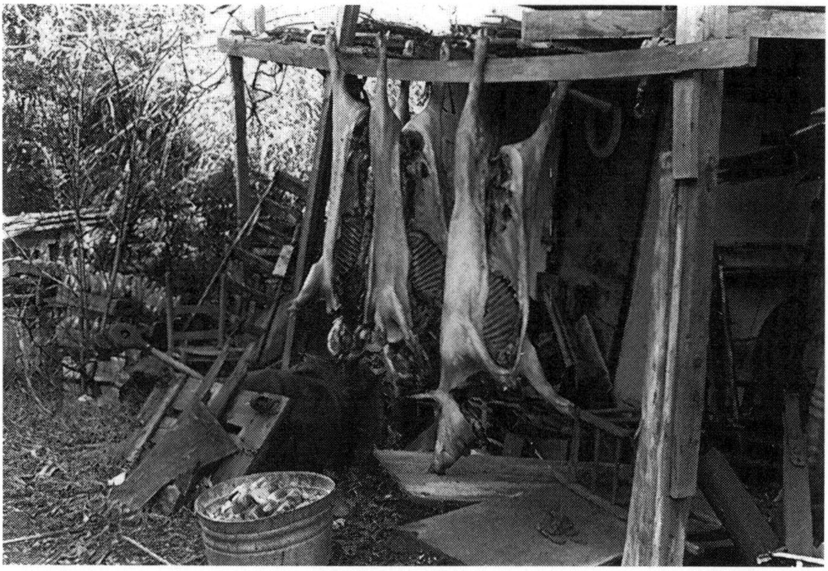

Photo © John Martin Taylor

Hog-killing in Tennessee

Maude was almost always called Old Maude, presumably because she had managed to live to the ripe old age of fourteen years when most of her peers would have long ago met an ignominious end at the local glue factory. She was a retired plow horse whose most valuable attribute (at least to a city kid suddenly in dire need of education in the ways of the farming life) was patience. She was patient to a fault. If I slipped from her bare back and landed beneath her feet, she just stopped in her tracks, looked around to be sure I was okay, and stood stock still as I tried awkwardly to remount her. Her patience no doubt spared me serious bodily harm that I would have suffered from a younger and more restless animal.

A major hurdle in the adjustment to farming life is getting comfortable with animals. All kinds of animals—chickens, pigs, cows, guinea fowls, etc. (not to mention the wild varieties that often showed up uninvited), as well as horses. I'm not sure where all those critters came from, but they suddenly appeared on the eighty-acre farm to which my father moved our completely city-bred family when I was twelve years old. He just ripped our roots from the two-bedroom house with running water and indoor plumbing that sat on a ragged quarter-acre lot in a pretty downtrodden area of East Nashville and plunked the entire family down on a small farm north of town. We moved into a ramshackle old house with five fireplaces (the only sources of heat), a tin roof, twelve-foot ceilings, tall skinny windows that rattled in the wind, a big front porch that overlooked the few tillable acres of creek bottom that would be our primary source of sustenance for the next few years, and no running water or indoor plumbing. It was the land that he loved. The house was not that important. He had probably grown up living in much less inviting structures.

My father grew up working the land cheek by jowl with black sharecroppers and other field hands on a big farm in Stewart County. As he described it, the farm was something of a post-Civil War stereotype—acres of fertile fields presided over by the big house, domicile of the gentleman farmer who suffered from an entrenched plantation mentality. The land was dotted with field hands' shacks that bore a haunting resemblance to the slave quarters they had replaced. My father probably lived in one of those during his formative years. Hauling in water for household use and relying on an outdoor privy for one's personal needs were familiar inconveniences he no doubt learned to tolerate during those years. They didn't seem to be that big of a deal to him.

It was the land—the landed experience and its potential—that enthralled him. And for reasons that I failed to fathom, my mother bought into the whole thing. She, too, was surprisingly knowledgeable in the ways of the farm and took to this new family experience with a vengeance. She planted a garden in a swath of creek bottom just next to the house and canned its produce during the long, hot summer afternoons, storing closets full of vegetables preserved for the winter months. She milked our lone Guernsey cow every morning and evening and churned butter from the rich milk characteristic of that breed. She delivered piglets, carting them in the winter from their hillside shed to the warmth of the kitchen fire to save their tiny lives. Each morning for breakfast she served biscuits made from scratch with freshly harvested eggs, just-churned Guernsey butter, and jam made from the blackberries she had picked from the briar patch that surrounded the lower creek bottom. And she somehow managed to get us ready for the school bus that came roaring down Pinhook Hill at the break of every weekday.

My father commuted to Nashville to keep his longstanding job as a city bus driver. He had enough seniority that he could choose what shift he wanted to work, and he usually chose the 3 p.m. to 11 p.m. shift so he could grab just a few winks after work and spend the days running the little farm and working the fields. I worked alongside him, learning the ropes. We planted enough acres of corn and hay to feed the pigs and cow with only a little supplement of commercial stock food (for some reason my father thought that small amounts of cotton seed meal were an important nutrient for farm animals). So, often side-by-side with my father as I entered tentatively into adolescence, I planted, chopped, cultivated, and eventually picked corn, raked and hauled hay, stacking it neatly around a tall pole, raking down the surface of the haystack to shed the rain, fed pigs and chickens and whatever other species was in need of food, slaughtered chickens for dinner, and helped castrate piglets (with no anesthesia and never in the dark of the moon), all under the careful eye of my land-loving father whose apparent goal was to live entirely off that land and what it bore.

For meat, we killed hogs. Hog-killing was something of a ritual, as well as the practical source of the meat course for the coming year's meals. My father presided, the high priest of hog killers, at least for our family. I think the role came naturally to him; he seemed to be a presider in a lot of situations although he often appeared uncomfortable in that role. But he was distinctly not uncomfortable at hog-killing. For that, he was in his element.

The event happened annually on Thanksgiving Day unless a fall warm spell made that day too warm to thoroughly cool the freshly slaughtered meat overnight. The most abiding experience of the ritual that I recall was the smell.

Early on Thanksgiving morning, my father loaded up the three hogs (always three, raised by us from their birth on food mostly from the produce of the creek bottom land that fronted the house) into the aging Ford pickup truck and took them a mile or so down Old Hickory Boulevard to where another local farmer had set up to kill the animals for the whole community. For a modest fee, he would stun the hogs with a .22-caliber rifle shot to the forehead, string them up by their back feet, slit their throat to allow them to bleed out, dunk the carcass in a vat of boiling water, and shave away the heat-loosened hair to reveal the pink-white remains of a hog carcass ready to be parceled into whatever parts the owner chose. My father would arrive back at the slaughtering area we had set up in our backyard, deposit the carcasses on a large temporary table-like structure, and then proceed to direct the ritual.

There is a smell to death, even purposeful death, of living organisms, and hogs, not generally noted for their pleasant odor even in life, are no exception. It was a haunting smell, a lingering chemosensory backdrop to the scene that doggedly persisted even in the face of the harsher odors of eviscerated internal organs and their contents and the nauseating emanations from the boiling cauldron of fat trimmed from the dissected carcasses being rendered into lard after squeezing out the last drops of oil from the residual bits of remaining skin. The skin-bits were called cracklings by the rural cognoscenti and were a major ingredient of crackling cornbread, a delicacy around hog-killing time that I never came to appreciate. Even now the memory of the smell of a big black cauldron of boiling fat is nauseating to me. I can still smell it, but I try not to. I also still don't like cornbread with or without cracklings.

The ritual took most of the day. My father eviscerated the carcasses and carved them up with surprising skill into their recognizably edible parts (hams, shoulders, side meat, jowls, etc.). He passed off the liver and lights (lungs), and maybe some other viscera, to my mother, who cooked them in another boiling cauldron for what seemed to me longer than necessary. The organs would later be cooled, ground up, and mushed into a heavily spiced loaf of something called *souse* that tasted terrible even if you hadn't watched it being made. It appeared to me that the main purpose of souse was to occupy a shelf in the refrigerator since I don't think I ever saw anyone eat any of it voluntarily.

As hog-killing day drew to a close—lard decanted into cast off Crisco tins, liver and lights set out to cool, neatly trimmed cuts of pork to be cured spread on the floor of the smokehouse to relinquish their final vestiges of life into the night—stiff fall air rising from the north promised a good night for cooling. The long and winding path from land to mouth was nearly over its final hurdle. There would be meat at our meals next year.

Vanilla Rock

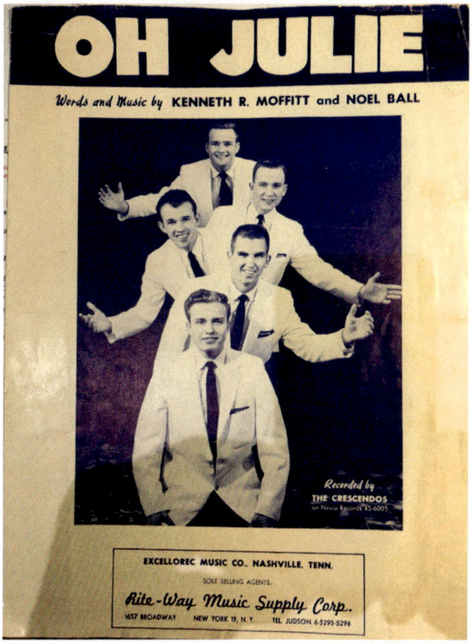

Author Memorabilia

In the year of our Lord nineteen hundred and fifty-eight, I was a member of a pop music quartet/quintet (the number varied) whose first record *Billboard* magazine proclaimed at one point the fifth most popular recording in the nation. The Crescendos … "Oh Julie" … Google it.

How in God's name did that happen? Another accident, I think. Certainly not a result of any gift of blinding talent on the part of anyone involved. We were just some ordinary guys in high school who liked the music and started fooling around with it, initially to put together an act for a school-sponsored "talent" show, the organizers of which interpreted "talent" very loosely. So loosely, in fact, that our little group won first prize. Had to be an accident. Without any shred of modesty, false or otherwise, I can assure you that the substance of our performance was anemic at its best, although we did a little better in the style department. However, buoyed by this unlikely award, we entered other high school talent shows in the city and won a second prize or two in the ones with the weaker lineup of acts—you know, baton twirlers, whistlers, tweenage girls, unshed baby fat ajiggle, attempting something they called modern dance, that sort of thing. Alongside that kind of talent, our renditions of The Platters' runaway hit, "The Great Pretender," and Marty Robbins's "A White Sport Coat and a Pink Carnation," sometimes fared better than they deserved.

In every city of any size in those days, the teenage music scene was dominated and often manipulated by a disc jockey who conducted a nightly show on AM radio where he spun forty-fives and took call-in requests, granting the requesters a minuscule sliver of fame by mentioning their names on the air. In Nashville, that person was Noel Ball (tag line, *Noel Ball Cigar and All*). Noel was probably close to forty, maybe five feet six with liberally pomaded hair slicked straight back. He was rarely seen absent his Churchill, well-chomped and almost always unlit, clamped in his mouth. Eventually, he also hosted a Saturday afternoon local TV show fashioned after the wildly popular nationally televised program, *American Bandstand*. Maybe he envisioned himself an emerging Dick Clark-like personality.

Noel Ball may not have shared the majority of Dick Clark's talents, but he was, like the boyish Philly hustler, an entrepreneur. The music scene at the time attracted many of that type. There was a lot of low-hanging fruit. It was about style, not substance. Panache trumped talent and there was a lot of money to be made. So, Noel Ball, like many of his compatriots across the country, trolled the local high school talent shows looking for acts that he thought had commercial potential. With the promise of a recording contract, he lured the acts that he thought had some promise into his web and then strung them along until he could figure out whether he could sell them to somebody in the music market with at least a smidgen of legitimacy. He latched on to us. We now called ourselves The Crescendos, and Noel promised that if we would just stick with him for a while, he would get us a shot at the big time. Probably to his surprise as well as ours, we did that and so did he.

This was 1958. This was Vanilla Rock—pre-Beatlemania, pre-promiscuous sex (well, mostly), pre-most of the currently popular drugs (there was booze and weed, but they were not easily available to young people under the age of twenty-one), just flirting with the phenomenon that was Elvis. I was only a few years from finally expanding my repertoire of emotional responses beyond uncontrolled weeping. Still being pretty careful.

But thirty one-nighters as an early act on Irving Feld's *The Biggest Show of Stars* was an education of sorts whether you were ready for it or not. The show was an assemblage of approximately fifty acts, beginning with a parade of one-hit wonders doing a song or two and concluding with the real stars—Frankie Avalon, LaVerne Baker, Jimmie Rodgers, Sam Cooke, the Everly Brothers, Jackie Wilson, and their ilk, the actual star on a given night varied —who would close the show sometime after midnight.

The show happened in a different city each night. A parade of decorated buses ferried us one-hit wonders (the big stars flew between dates) to the next city starting after the close of that day's show. We would arrive at the new city in the wee hours, check into a hotel, sleep for a bit, and then meet at the assigned venue in the afternoon for rehearsal with the orchestra. There were a few hours between rehearsal and the actual performance when *The Biggest Show of Stars* was repeated and we were loaded up on buses and carted off to the next show town. This was the routine for a full month. It was one of the most disorienting and exhausting periods of my young life. There was precious little glamour in it. Any such fantasies rapidly dissipated in the face of the stark reality.

But there was the odd, enlightening vignette. For example, in a city the name of which I do not remember (in my memory this month was an amalgam of cities with no defining borders), for the first time in my young life, I beheld a naked woman. Lillie Storey was one-half of The Storey Sisters whose song, "Bad Motorcycle" (leaning heavily on onomatopoeia—*budn, budn, budn*), was popular enough (along with the fact that they were strikingly lovely young women) that they landed on *The Biggest Show of Stars* doing their thing in the spot just preceding the Crescendos. On this particular night we waited off-stage as usual during the Storey Sisters' act ready to enter the limelight as soon as they exited. When finished, Lillie Storey walked off-stage directly in front of where we waited. She paused a moment and slid the thin straps of her gown from her shoulders, the dress pooling around her slim ankles. Underneath the dress she wore only a very scant pair of totally transparent panties. She looked at us, smiled, tossed the gown over her shoulder, and sauntered off nonchalantly toward the dressing rooms. I was speechless. I had no time to digest that existential moment as the emcee was announcing the entrance of the Crescendos. The show must go on, any maturing experiences of adolescence transpiring around the periphery of the action be damned!

Fortunately, I think, the whole thing was over in a year, probably about par for the course for one-hit wonders at the time. But what a year it should have been! Picture it. A young man at the peak of adolescence. Juices fully revved. Far away from any mitigating forces—family, school, church, reasonably sane and level-headed adults—touring the width and breadth of North America in the company of strangers most of whom seemed primarily interested in indulging the desires of the flesh for which there were ample opportunities. All the makings of a crash course in how the real world worked and how its inhabitants conducted themselves in the day-to-day business of getting life done. Ah, what a year it should have been.

I think the reason that this overdose of worldliness didn't take was that the entire situation contrasted so enormously with anything I had been aware of before leaping (or being thrown by a conspiracy of opportunity and social pressure) naked and hopelessly naïve into the deepest end of the roiling pool of human experience. I had to marshal all of my energy against the threat of being captured by the powerful undertow and ferried off to a destination that I dared not contemplate. So, those sturdy flotation devices that had been carefully woven by the dedicated efforts of parents and some other people who cared about me into my perception of whom I was saved the day. Such concepts instilled early on endure. Some years later, a trio of musically inclined young men admonished us to "Teach your children well ..." But be careful what you teach them. One does not readily unlearn.

Performing for the Church of the Ambivalent Word

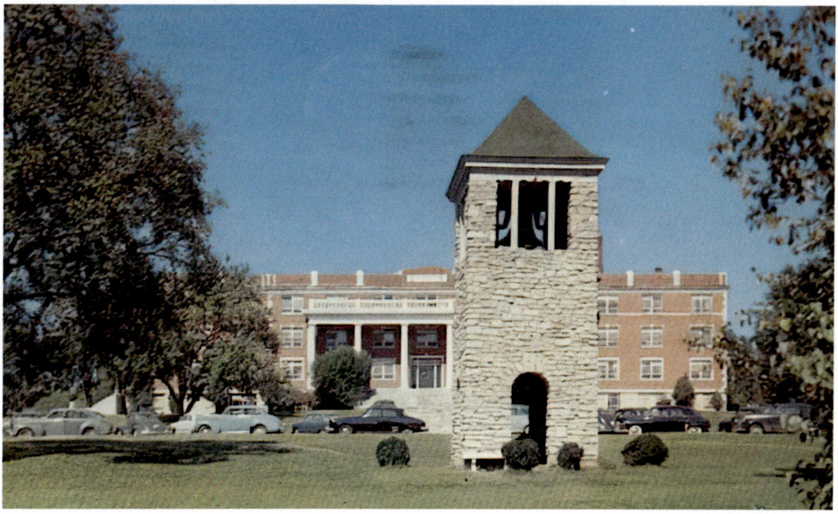

Vintage Postcard

David Lipscomb College

The New Testament author known as Saint John alluded metaphorically to the eternity and nature of the incarnate Jesus as the *Word.* "In the beginning was the Word...." he wrote at the start of his gospel. My parents and many of their acquaintances professed to believe that, not just the metaphor, but all of the actual words as found mostly in the King James Bible. They did what they could to indoctrinate that notion into their children with varying degrees of success. Practically from the time I could walk and talk, I was their star pupil.

If your experience at the time was bounded by the geography of Nashville and its environs, you could easily believe that the dominant religious institution in the world was a loosely organized fundamentalist entity that called itself the Church of Christ. The "Church" had no organized hierarchy. It was a collection of autonomous congregations of people who held a narrow spectrum of views, anchored by a conviction that the Bible was the literal word of God and was the sole, unerring guide to a pretty uncompromising way of life. Although its theology has evolved since then, at the time it was not long on the doctrine of grace, and its spokesmen—all men, mostly self-appointed—were fond of Bible-thumping harangues with frighteningly graphic descriptions of a seething, brimstone-fueled hell.

Somewhere along their way, my parents had fallen in thrall to the Church of Christ, and it became the primary social as well as religious experience of our family. I bought the whole thing, swallowed it hook, line, and sinker. I was too insecure to do otherwise. I discovered that I had some talent for performing in public which I could summon to demonstrate my convictions. I think now that my youthful religious experience was more the performance than a soul-wrenching passion for that brand of Christianity. I have often relied more on perception than reality in a lot of life's important matters. Although that has served me well as a pragmatic strategy, I don't think it has made me a better person.

The flagship educational institution of the Church of Christ was David Lipscomb College (now a university), a small private college located on the south edge of town with tentacles reaching deep into the hinterlands from which it retrieved students who arrived on campus steeped in the relevant dogma, anxious to deepen those convictions, and equally anxious to find someone to marry who shared their faith. At least those seemed to be the prime motivations for most Lipscomb students at the time. I am sure that there was also a roiling undercurrent of adolescent ids, fed by the church's strict sexual attitudes, but nobody dared talk about such things: dress codes were carefully followed; public displays of affection were anathema; no drinking or dancing; church services were attended at least two and preferably three times per week; and chapel services and Bible classes were daily requirements.

I was the first person in my family to attend college. A good student, I was encouraged by teachers and some more perceptive family members to extend my education. My only realistic choice was Lipscomb; since money was scarce, an offer of a scholarship confirmed that fact. Although there may have been adolescent rumblings of religious ambivalence beginning before then, it was on the campus of the Church of Christ's flagship institution of higher learning, that the inconsistencies became hauntingly clear. There were many. The Word was not as reliable as I had been led to believe.

I found it impossible to accept the fundamental premise that the Bible's words were descended literally from the heavens and intended as the infallible truth about the purpose and nature of the human condition. For one thing, some serious mental gymnastics were required to explain apparent contradictions in the holy text. But that didn't seem to be a major issue for the people in control.

There was also the difficulty reconciling the biblical version of the purpose and nature of life with the subject matter of biology, the academic area that most interested me. I found the King James Bible woefully deficient as a source of accurate information about either human biology or the human condition in general. Even my science teachers couldn't always conceal their discomfort at attempting to balance their convictions on the knife-edge boundary between unerring commitment to the teachings of the "Church" and the often-contradictory corpus of scientific truth. It was hard to reconcile the two. I didn't think anyone had figured that out and I wasn't entirely sure that they had tried very hard.

And then there were the *open secrets*. These people who maintained that their salvation depended on strict adherence to the biblical formula often behaved otherwise. And everybody knew that. There was illicit sex, homosexuality (an abomination, thundered many a Sunday sermonizer with a hearty thump of the good book), alcoholism, and a lot of other behaviors that belied the Sunday morning proclamations. Even some church leaders led undisclosed private lives that were only murmured about in hushed tones by ill-willed gossipmongers but that everybody knew about—open secrets. I think that's what happens when you try to force inherently unruly human beings into such a restrictive mold—you create fertile ground for nurturing ambivalence.

But I tried, at least for a while, victim of my own need to please people I cared about. I even took up preaching at a little country church near Shelbyville for a bit. It was a congregation of wonderfully warm and caring folks, mostly families of small farms, who were gracious to a fault. But I was convinced that they were not getting fair value for the few dollars they paid me each Sunday. I just put my check back into the collection plate. I was performing and didn't think I was doing an especially good job of it. Try as I might, my heart just wasn't in it.

Upon reflection from this distant vantage point, I am amazed at how deeply and for how long my family's religion influenced my life. I guess that's what religion does if you take it seriously. Marriage is an example of what I mean. Thoroughly committed to the rule that sexual intercourse was to be limited to a single, lifelong relationship, I married the wrong woman when I was too young to know better. I remained in that marriage for more than thirty years before finally facing up to the reality that I'd made a mistake. During that time, I mostly escaped into a successful and demanding career rather than deal with the relevant personal issues. That was sufficient to keep up appearances that were convincing enough to satisfy my family and the people whose favor they valued. I suppose the reality of that relationship was one of those open secrets that were essential to the fragile integrity of adherents of the Church of the Ambivalent Word.

There was one spectacular reward for my efforts. The birth of my only child, a beautiful, gifted, loving, and genuinely human daughter, in the wee small hours of a fateful day in San Francisco in the early seventies changed my world forever. I still marvel at that. Thank you, Heather, for being you.

Becoming

Wonderbilt

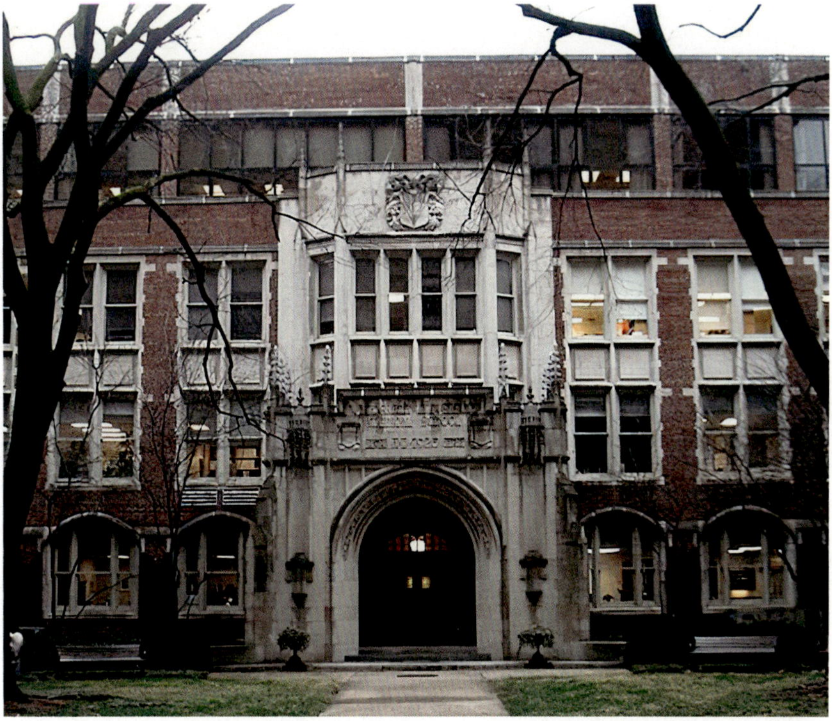

Reid Sullivan/Wikimedia Commons

Vanderbilt University School of Medicine

There were two letters in the mailbox on a summer morning when my life took a direction that I would not have believed possible. One letter informed me that I had been accepted by the University of Tennessee College of Medicine and that I would be awarded a full scholarship there. The other letter was from Vanderbilt School of Medicine, surely a gentle message that I had not been accepted at that august institution but that the admissions committee wished me well. I was ready for that message. Acceptance and a scholarship awaiting me in Memphis, I was perfectly happy to let the unlikely dream of an elite medical education at Vanderbilt recede in my rearview mirror as I moved on to just get the job done and then see what happened next.

To their everlasting credit, the gray-bearded traditionalists on the admissions committee at Vanderbilt didn't let me off so easily. To my surprise, the second letter informed me that I was also accepted for admission to Vanderbilt. There was no mention of financial help, though, and money was a big issue for me. Standing there in a bright morning sun, a letter in each hand, I felt suspended between the equal and opposite forces of the practicality of the situation and the chance to realize an impossible dream—dangling precariously over what felt like a bottomless chasm between the irresistible forces of my head and my heart.

I'm not sure where I summoned the audacity to even apply to medical school at Vanderbilt. Those prized positions were reserved for well-off graduates of elite East Coast universities—Harvard, Princeton, Yale, the usual suspects—who arrived in their vintage BMWs and sauntered confidently onto campus like the children of privilege whom they were. Although my life to date had been spent almost within a stone's throw of the west Nashville campus, I had always thought of Vanderbilt as a remote wonderland of academic sophistication, accessible only to the children of the moneyed and well-connected. What was a poor kid from a hardscrabble truck farm north of town, graduate of an undistinguished small college that existed primarily to propagate a marginal fundamentalist religion, doing with such aspirations? Get a life, Ken Brigham! For God's sake, take what they give you and make the best of it. *Don't look a gift horse in the mouth,* my father might have said.

I sat near the back of the medical amphitheater overlooking the steeply tiered rows of fellow freshman Vanderbilt medical students, trying hard to suppress the palpitations that jack-hammered in my chest and to look like I belonged there. We were waiting for the dean to appear and welcome us to what would be the most demanding four years that any of us had undertaken thus far.

I was there because of my older sister, Elizabeth, and her husband, Bill (still known even in his later years as Junior) Hill. Although neither of them had attended college, they insisted that

I go to Vanderbilt and volunteered to help with the finances if need be. I'm not sure why they did that, why they valued Vanderbilt over the state university. Maybe I telegraphed that attitude without being aware of it or maybe the reputation of Nashville's premier university influenced even people who had no way to judge such institutions objectively. Whatever their reasons, that decision changed the subsequent course of my life. Over those next four years, I felt for the first time the inexplicable thrill of discovery and built a long and happy career free dancing nimbly along that path.

I believe that the principal factor that distinguishes educational institutions like Harvard from North Louisiana State Teachers College (if there is such a school) is the strength of an intangible asset that I'll call the *academic aura*. It is the power of that invisible magnet that attracts students, faculty, alumni donations, government and foundation grant dollars, and the attention of the academic power brokers, all the things that you need to establish and sustain the brand.

Those things may well influence the value of an institution's proffered education, but not uniformly so. It all depends on what the school intends to do and on the student. Was my medical education superior to what I would have experienced at UT? I'm not sure about that. It may well be that I would have emerged from that institution better prepared to care for the infirmities of my fellows than I did (that medical school was very good at generating competent doctors well-prepared to meet the medical needs of its state's citizens), but I believe it unlikely that I would have been so captivated by the thrill of discovery, the heartbeat of an institution founded on and sustained by research. Approaching those divergent paths from a vantage point in Memphis, I might well have danced off in a different direction.

After forays into several other elite medical institutions, I returned to Vanderbilt where I spent almost thirty years basking in the glow of the institution's academic aura and free dancing along the exhilarating path of scientific discovery. Who would have imagined that I would be admitted into the sacred space of unbridled imagination that thrived in the protected confines of the academic ivory tower? I would not have dared anticipate that possibility.

My father wanted me to become a Railway Express Agent. I hope he would not be disappointed.

Enlightenment in Baltimore

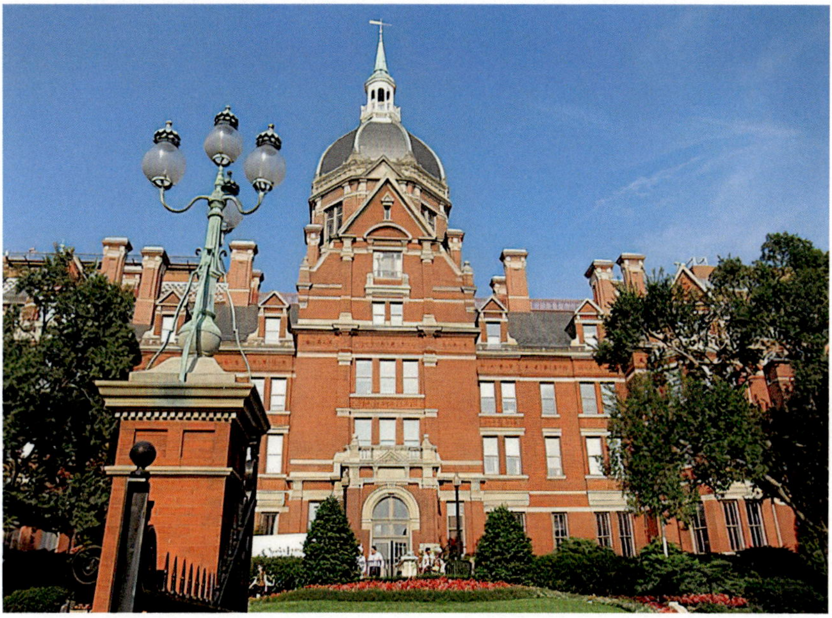

The Johns Hopkins Hospital

If you were looking for a residency upon graduating from medical school in the mid-sixties, you would soon realize that the perceived academic value of such a position was inversely proportional to any serious gestures to the niceties of medical practice. Big city hospitals that delivered no-frills care to mainly uninsured indigent people—Grady in Atlanta, Charity (The Big Free) in New Orleans, San Francisco General, et al.—were popular. At the top of that list was the venerable Osler Medical Service at Johns Hopkins Hospital, legacy of Sir William Osler, the consensus godfather of modern American medicine. Every year, freshly minted medical graduates from across the country, hoping to illuminate their CVs in the reflected glow of its iconic namesake's aura, competed for the few internship slots on the Hopkins Osler Service.

The more difficult and uncomfortable those coveted positions were, the more they seemed to attract the best and brightest candidates. Difficulty and discomfort were somehow conflated with academic rigor, and the powers that be at Hopkins had, over the years, perfected the seamless integration of difficulty and discomfort into an unrivaled educational experience.

There was record heat in Baltimore the summer I arrived there. The Osler Service resided in an unairconditioned red brick building anchored to its spot facing North Broadway by the accumulated historic weight of an iconic dome. The several floors of mostly open wards simmered in the triple-digit heat, basting the rows of nearly naked patients in their own juices and mercilessly roasting the white-clad interns like Christmas turkeys as they bustled about their duties. This was heat that was difficult to ignore. There were rigors in the frontline trenches where one learned to wrestle effectively with the blood and guts of medical reality and if you wanted the education, you just had to grit your teeth and deal with the rigors.

There was also the call schedule, no doubt designed by a closet sadist determined to saddle these naively idealistic young people with the disorienting consequences of sleep deprivation. Interns were on call twenty-four hours a day for six and a half days each week. The primary responsibility for newly admitted patients was assigned to whomever was next in line, regardless of when the admission occurred or of any consideration of the severity of the new patient's immediate problem. So, subject to the biopathologic whims of the citizens of East Baltimore, an intern could end up with a series of admissions and urgent medical demands happening in the wee small hours that precluded any biologically plausible attempt to satisfy one's need for sleep. Whether Osler ever said or wrote, "You don't learn medicine at home in bed," is not clear, but that dictum was attributed to him by the distinguished Hopkins faculty dedicated to educating the next generation of medical leaders, and it was frequently "quoted" as justification for the truly barbaric demands they made of their ambitious charges.

But difficulty and discomfort be damned, my time at Hopkins was the most intense and exciting revelation of the realities of my chosen profession that I would ever have the fortitude and good fortune to survive. Toiling day and night at the bedsides of unfortunate and often careless people in desperate efforts to prolong lives that did not seem especially concerned about longevity, I learned both the art and science of healing. The long shadows of one of the most distinguished medical faculties in the world splayed over those Osler wards, captivating a rising generation of their kind with the passion that drove their efforts to illuminate the realities of human biology and to use that knowledge to care for their sick brethren. Sitting at the humble bedsides of often penniless East Baltimoreans in the shadows of living medical giants and under the careful watch of Sir William Osler's ghost is where I became a doctor.

Since then, the mentality that led to postgraduate medical training deliberately designed as a test of survival has mercifully yielded to a saner, more rational, and almost certainly more effective approach. We've come to recognize that while you may not learn medicine at home in bed, neither do you learn anything very well when exhausted, and exhaustion is a moral hazard when your actions have life or death consequences.

In the small hours of a hot July day, Sir William's ghost must still haunt the now-air-conditioned patient units in the ever-expanding complex of buildings fronting North Broadway and adjacent East Baltimore streets. He surely keeps a keen eye on the doings of each new crop of aspiring medical graduates that arrives there every summer. Okay, let them get the rest they need to be at their best, but keep their noses hard against the grindstone of demands that their profession will make of them for as long as they practice it. This is where they'll learn to deal with those demands. This is where they have a fighting chance to begin to master the art and science of the life-consuming vocation they have chosen. If their teachers choose the right pupils and do their jobs, this is still where doctors are made.

India and the Solid Geometry of Our Planet

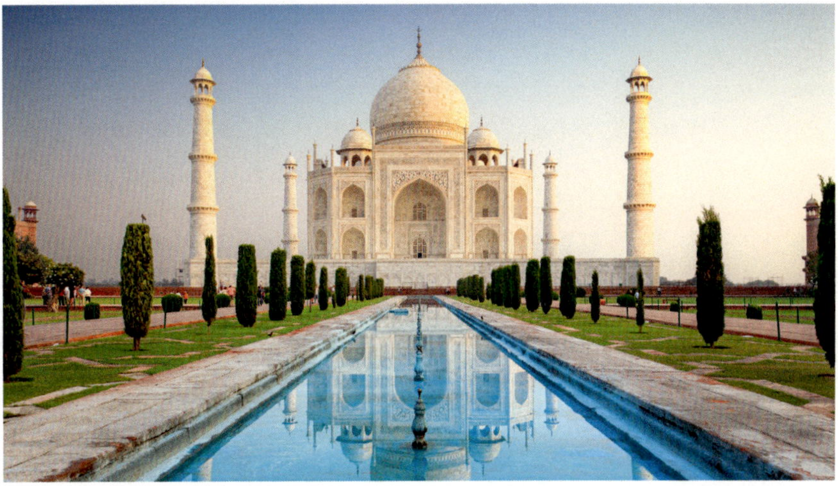

Sean Hsu/Adobe Photo

The Taj Mahal, Agra, India

To dispel any possible thoughts you may have had to the contrary, let me assure you that, at least in the year 1968, the planet on which we dwell was a globe, or some shape approximating that description. I know that for a fact. I had the special opportunity to circumnavigate the planet during that year and had the earth been flat, I would now be floating weightless somewhere in the cosmic ether, having dropped off the edge probably in the vicinity of the Indian Ocean as I wended my way from Baltimore through Europe to Calcutta and then back to Baltimore via the Far East.

Why Calcutta? Because that's where the cholera was.

How the venerable Johns Hopkins medical institution, seedbed for the current era of scientific medicine, became interested in cholera, eventually establishing a cholera research unit in the Calcutta Infectious Disease Hospital to which two of their medical residents each year (myself and David Fedson in 1968) were sent to assist during the cholera season, is interesting. It was an accident. Or at least the (possibly apocryphal) tale certainly sounds that way.

Here is the tale as I learned it. Charles C.J. (Chuck) Carpenter, completing his stint as brilliant and legendary Chief Resident on the vaunted Osler Medical Service at Hopkins, decided that he was interested in kidney diseases (nephrology) as a subspecialty. Although cholera was not common in the United States, and was mainly a gastrointestinal disease, he became fascinated with reports that the kidneys of many patients with that disease stopped doing their job. And a lot of those people died as a result. Dr. Carpenter was a very smart and curious man and knew that often something essential can be learned from such an unexpected association of bodily malfunctions. A lot of people in India got cholera, and it so happened that Hopkins had a small Johns Hopkins Center for Medical Research and Training (JHCMRT) in Calcutta.

Chuck and a few associates packed up a bunch of equipment for doing dialysis, a last-ditch approach to treating kidney failure, and headed halfway around the world to figure this thing out. What they discovered was that cholera didn't affect the kidneys at all. The cause of renal failure in patients with cholera was dehydration, a consequence of the loss of prodigious amounts of fluid by diarrhea. If you replaced the fluid as rapidly as it was lost, patients lived and the kidneys were just fine. Get an IV going as soon as possible and pour in the fluid and within minutes the near-comatose and pulseless patient was sitting up smiling and rattling off something in Bengali that sounded positive. The death rate from cholera in the Calcutta Infectious Disease Hospital plummeted almost overnight from double digits to near zero in the Hopkins unit. The dialysis equipment collected dust in a storeroom someplace and Dr. C.C.J. Carpenter made a professional U-turn and became a specialist in infectious diseases. His work in Calcutta helped to establish a cholera research unit there that became a hotbed of basic and clinical discoveries that over ensuing years added to the corpus of medical knowledge at many levels and developed practical approaches to fluid and electrolyte replacement that continue to this day to save lives.

So a complicated set of accidents was responsible for my arriving at the Gateway to India on the Bombay waterfront (this was pre-Mumbai), jostling my way through a cloying mass of beggars, snake charmers, pimps, food vendors, tour guides, and sellers of other goods and services that I did not wish to know about, toward the entrance to the truly grand Taj Mahal Palace Hotel. I mean truly grand!

Upon this first introduction to India, I was assaulted with the mind-bending reality of intimately juxtaposed contrasts so enormous that stepping across the threshold of the Taj Mahal Hotel felt like taking Alice's hand and passing, in an instant, through the looking glass. Such shocking juxtapositions came to define my experience of India. The society of that country was composed of parallel universes as different in composition and texture as it is possible to be. From the waterfront promenade throbbing with the *sturm und drang* of the darker human passions, I was suddenly transported into a marble and gold festooned wonderland of quiet dignity, elegantly costumed and graciously accommodating servants of my every wish, and opulent accommodations the likes of which I could not have imagined. I soaked for a while in a marble tub in a bathroom larger than my apartment in Baltimore and contemplated that other world just beyond the granite fortress of the Taj.

On the night of November 26, 2008, a hail of terrorists' gunfire shattered that fragile looking glass barrier between opulence and squalor that protected the Taj Majal Palace Hotel from the teeming mass of desperate humanity surrounding it. Probably inevitable. We do not sustain such side-by-side inequities forever. There is no wall strong enough. We are, after all, all of us, human.

Ah, the Taj. The real one, I mean. I visited Agra, home to the Taj Mahal and was smitten even more forcefully with the reality of a fragile barrier that seemed everywhere to impose itself, if tentatively, between grinding poverty and mesmerizing beauty. What separated the two was at once enormous, impenetrable, and deceptively brittle, barely sufficient to maintain its integrity. The beggars and hustling guides who congregated outside the opulent marble and precious stone inlaid gate leading to the inner sanctum of the Taj knew their boundaries. They were not permitted beyond the gate, and they respected that limitation. One could imagine that if they chose, their mere mass could easily breach the restriction, but they probably knew that respecting the perimeter was essential to their survival, likely essential to the social integrity of the entire country at the time.

One need only to pass through the bejeweled gate to experience what I am convinced is one of the most transcendentally beautiful vistas that human beings have managed to create. A long reflecting pool. The lightning-white marble and precious stone inlaid façade of the tomb standing erect at the distal end of the pool, proudly admiring its reflection. There is a marble bench just at the front of the pool. John and Jackie Kennedy sat there once, no doubt as thrilled by the spectacle as was I. I sat there for a long time.

Not a rail-thin hustling Indian in sight. They were poised outside the gate, on the other side of the invisible wall, waiting for the travelers to do the deed, recover from their bout of sensory overload, and emerge back into reality, perhaps more pliable than when they had arrived in Agra, hot, tired, and dusty from the trip. Those gaunt Indians and their darker side of reality were as real and permanent a part of the landscape as the inner sanctum of the Taj.

Calcutta was a smell before it was a place. The propeller-driven twin-engine airplane made two false passes over the landing strip to frighten off the cows lolling about there before setting down with a jarring thud and bouncing jauntily for a way along a potholed former military airstrip. The plane rattled to a stop beside a corrugated iron structure that looked more like an abandoned warehouse than an airport. Immediately upon descending the steps to the tarmac, I was introduced without preamble to the odor of Calcutta.

It was a unique olfactory experience. Were it not so searingly harsh, it wouldn't have been an especially unpleasant smell. Earthy, for sure, but I wasn't nauseated, just shocked by the intensity. The smell of Calcutta was a blend of burning dung patties (fuel for the roadside makeshift cooking stoves that were everywhere), simmering mixtures of pungent spices (oozing the scent of exorbitant amounts of cumin), the emanations from teeming masses of human bodies roasting in the merciless tropical sun, and probably contributions from a thousand other anonymous plants, animals, and decaying organic matter. You may think that sounds like your worst possible olfactory nightmare, but it wasn't really. I remember it more like the aroma of a very overripe cheese, a smell that has an appeal for some of us. That's about as good a comparison as I can muster, but there was no simile that did the odor of Calcutta justice. It was unique.

After an interminable taxi ride which exceeds my ability to describe, I was welcomed on my arrival at the New Kenilworth Hotel by Rajan Xavier, a Bengali who allegedly assumed that name after converting to Catholicism and, I suspect, because of his desire to identify more closely with the mainly Western guests of the hotel that he managed. He was conscientious and good at his job. For the next couple of months, this British-style boarding hotel was where I lived, slept, sometimes took afternoon tea, and ate. Meals were in a common room and there was a repetitive menu that cycled weekly. I remember a lot of boiled meat with boiled potatoes. I distinctly remember that boiled goat (likely from an animal that had otherwise outlived its usefulness) was served on Tuesdays when we would repair to the Kwality Diner, just a short walk into town, for a delicious meal of authentic Indian food, none of which, as best I could tell, was boiled.

So much for the travelogue. There is a lot more, but I wasn't there on Johns Hopkins's (and indirectly the U.S. government's) rupee just to enjoy the view. My reason for being there and the core of my Indian experience took place in a three-story concrete building with big open rectangular holes in the walls (hardly qualifying as windows) overlooking a large plot of land the principal functions of which seemed to be as a repository for coconut shells tossed from the building after being drained of their milk by the cholera patients inside, and as a pasture for several dozen goats. Welcome to the Calcutta Infectious Disease Hospital.

For the next couple of months, I spent each day there rehydrating to life people near death from cholera and participating in several research projects, some of which resulted in the development of oral solutions of water and electrolytes that could substitute for intravenous fluids and so could be given anywhere. The significance of that is enormous. Eventually thousands of people who would have died of dehydration in the remote villages where cholera was rampant and hospitals were rare would live. That experience was one of the great privileges of my life. I didn't plan it that way. Nobody did. I was there pretty much by accident.

Research leading to life-saving advances in medicine is not always glamorous or complicated. Envision this: A large open room with cholera cots (bare cots with a hole at anus level covered by a rubber sheet with an opening strategically designed to align with the hole in the mattress) lining the room cheek by jowl, separated from one another by only a few inches. Beneath the ten beds comprising the Hopkins Unit were yellow plastic buckets with gradations in deciliters marked on their sides with magic marker. Patients to be evaluated for oral replacement were resuscitated with intravenous fluids on arrival (otherwise they would have died) and then had a tube placed through the nose into the stomach and attached to a reservoir of fluid suspended above the bed. My job (and David Fedson's) was to make rounds every hour, record the level of fluid in the container beneath the bed and adjust the rate of fluid entering the stomach tube to equal the previous hour's output. A simple concept: input equals output. The definition of a steady state (homeostasis, if you like), a ubiquitous phenomenon essential to normal bodily functions of humans and other living things. Do enough of those studies and you will see whether the fluid you are using to rehydrate these patients was working, whether you could forego the IVs.

But what was the fluid? Here's where we learn (if we didn't already know it) that concepts that appear too simple often are. The composition of the replacement fluid was based on basic research on how fluids are absorbed by the gastrointestinal tract, and the discovery in the process that cholera was almost exclusively a secretory disease. Absorption by the gut was essentially normal, including the enhanced absorption that resulted from the presence of sugar. So a fluid was designed with sugar as well as sodium, potassium and all the other things that were being depleted by the secretory side of the equation. The idea was that if you just flooded the gut with the stuff, it could absorb enough to overcome what was being lost and you could keep the situation stable until the effects of the cholera toxin wore off and win both the battle and the war of fluid dynamics. And indeed that turned out to be the case. It wasn't elegant. It wasn't pretty. It wasn't complicated. But it worked.

A Day in the Foreshadow of the Prize

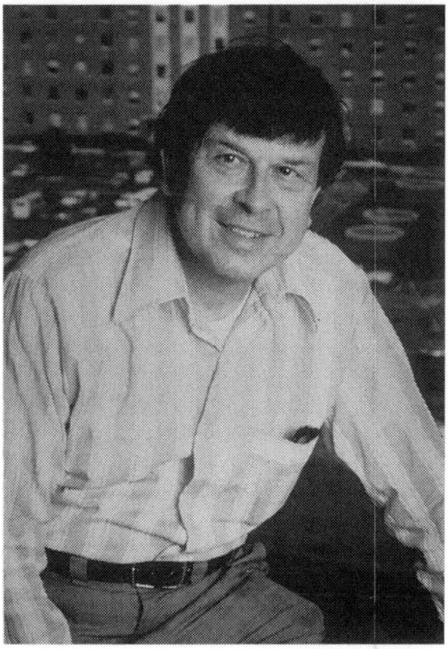

Wikimedia Commons

Carleton Gajdusek, Nobel laureate 1976

1968

The one-thousand nine-hundred sixty-eighth year of the Common Era and ninth year of the sixties, when a seismic tremor of social disquiet threatened to dismantle the grand American experiment, was not a good time to be exposed to the whims of a government in dire need of rediscovering its moral compass. Martin Luther King, Jr. and Bobby Kennedy were both assassinated that year. Opposition to the Asian war was rampant. American soldiers massacred scores of innocent civilians at My Lai. Yippies took on the Chicago police at the Democratic National Convention. Eventually, Lyndon Johnson was forced by the accumulating weight of his nation's misdeeds to cancel plans to run for president. And I and my peers were just moving from medical residencies to the front of the queue of anxious young medics facing a couple of years of enforced servitude in some branch of the armed services. Precious few of us relished that prospect. A limited number of positions in the U.S. Public Health Service Commissioned Corps (a barely legitimate branch of the armed services) was as painless a way as possible to do your time at a safe distance from physical danger. If the cards fell right, Carleton Gajdusek might be my ticket through the two-year service obligation to whatever was to happen next.

Paul Brown was a wiry, handsome veteran of a stint at the National Institutes of Health when he came to Hopkins to complete his formal medical training. More than a little vain, he spent a lot of time by the pool, the fortified centerpiece of the housing complex where residents and their families lived, carefully nurturing his near-perfect tan. He performed well enough as a resident, which he probably viewed essentially as a necessary evil, a brief interlude before returning to Gadjusek's laboratory at the NIH and resuming his real career interest in diseases of "unconventional viruses."

Because escaping the war was at the top of my list of priorities, I had committed to a Public Health Service position at the Center for Disease Control (the *and Prevention* was added later), but for those of us with an academic bent, the prime spots for insulating oneself from the threat of armed conflict while doing something constructive were at the NIH. I had not been particularly friendly with Paul Brown, but he must have learned somehow that I would really like to do my obligatory service time in Bethesda. And there must have been some element of the Hopkins communal spirit that, aware of some spots available in Gadjusek's lab, caused Paul to interrupt his afternoon sun time to arrange a day for me with Dr. Gajdusek to feel out the possibility of joining his lab.

On my first visit to the Bethesda campus of the NIH, I found my way to what was then the National Institute for Neurological Diseases and Blindness and to a small, cluttered laboratory presided over by a casually dressed, boyish fellow whose Beatle-oid mop of dark hair fell across his face as he bent over something on his desk that appeared to command his rapt attention. When he finally looked up, responding to my repeated efforts to announce my presence by making a series of guttural sounds and pacing nervously about the room, the questioning glare of his penetrating dark eyes stopped me dead in my tracks. He said nothing for a moment. I had the feeling that he was trying to remember who I was and what I was doing there. For a few seconds, I wondered the same thing. Eventually Dr. Gajdusek appeared to figure things out and was a gracious host during a memorable afternoon.

My enduring impression from that brief brush with the man who would be awarded a Nobel Prize in less than a decade for his pioneering work with kuru, an obscure brain disease unique to the North Fore people in New Guinea, was his maps. Gajdusek had become so enamored of the obscure people who lived on that scattering of Micronesian islands that he moved there for a while and learned the language. Realizing that there were no maps of many of the islands, Gajdusek, apparently a brilliant polymath (he studied physics, biology, chemistry, and mathematics as an undergraduate), took up cartography and produced the only existing detailed maps of much of the area. His original hand drawings, kept in several bound notebooks resting in a protected space on a laboratory shelf, were works of art.

Dr. Gajdusek carefully removed the notebooks from the shelf and spread them out on a lab bench, obviously inviting me to admire them. I had the feeling that he was as proud of those lovely documents as he was of the groundbreaking science that would bring him the ultimate recognition of the Nobel. I did not need to feign admiration for his truly extraordinary handiwork, but I couldn't think of anything to say that would do them justice. I was awed by this extraordinary man whose boundless intellect fed with such apparent ease a reservoir of curiosity about the world and its inhabitants that was contemptuous of any constraints that his chosen profession might have expected of him.

In my limited experience (I've had some contact with three of them), Nobel laureates are an unlikely lot. Gajdusek was no exception. How does the Yonkers-born son of a Hungarian butcher navigate the rarely trod path through Harvard Med School, postdocs at Columbia, Cal Tech, and Harvard, and to the Walter and Eliza Hall Institute of Medical Research in Melbourne, Australia? Apart from the fact that he was a virologist and found himself in that part of the world, why New Guinea, why the obscure North Fore people and why kuru, not typical of viral infections of the brain? I'll lay you favorable odds that the whole scenario was a cosmic accident. I suspect that people, places, events unfolded in Gajdusek's life according to no plan of his or any life-guiding force. They just happened. I think Dr. Gajdusek free danced his way along an ill-defined path that happened to take him to Stockholm.

Carleton Gajdusek was awarded the Nobel Prize in Physiology or Medicine in 1976. He had connected kuru with the ritualistic consumption of relatives' brains by the Fore people and had transmitted the disease to chimpanzees by injecting their brains with homogenates of brain samples from Fore men who had the disease. He recognized kuru's very long incubation time and inferred that it was infectious although devoid of inflammation, a theretofore universal characteristic of viral brain diseases. He made the connection to Creutzfeldt-Jakob disease and similar human neurodegenerative disorders. Later, the Nobel Committee rewarded work by others who discovered a new class of infectious agents called *prions* that were the causative agents of the diseases that preoccupied Gajdusek throughout his career.

I was offered the position at the NIH and would have jumped at the chance, but the CDC would not free me of the earlier commitment that I had made to them. Another of those forks in the road that could have taken me in a very different direction but didn't, for reasons that were surely just random consequences of humans behaving like humans.

The Grand Canyon on an Ass

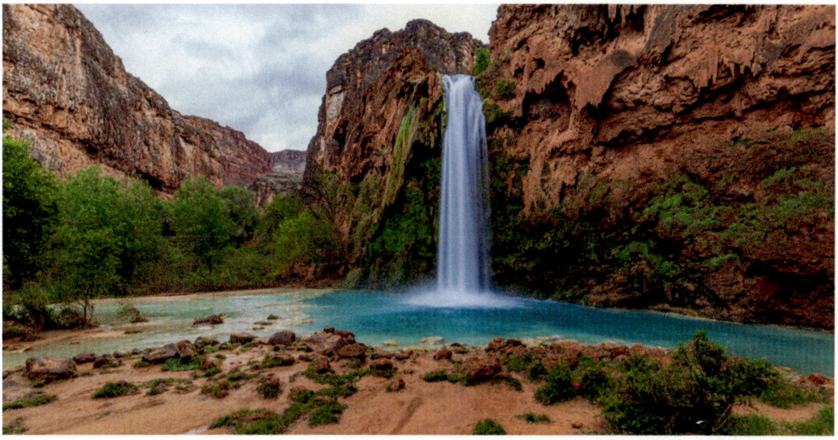

Michael Whitworth/Adobe Photo

Supai Falls

The drive from where we left the Route 66 pavement heading to the site at the south rim of the Grand Canyon that was the jumping off place for access to the ancestral home of the Havasupai Nation on the canyon floor was seventy miles long. It seemed longer.

Sunlight angled across the desolate high plateau on a crisp, fall morning. The government Jeep from the Indian Health Service (IHS) motor pool wasn't built for comfort and more than lived up to that reputation as we flounced our way for miles on a rutted track toward the canyon lip. We had shipped provisions in advance to the little clapboard one-nurse clinic that served as the sole medical facility for the majestic home of the noble Havasupai. We had also arranged to be met at the canyon rim by a native with his few shabby but allegedly sure-footed mules to escort us and our remaining supplies down the precarious hours-long switchback path to the bottom of one of our world's most grand natural sites. Except for the services of a skilled helicopter pilot, that was the only way to get there. Government rates wouldn't pay for a helicopter ride. Even the U.S. mail was delivered there by mule train.

I was the only doctor on the small team charged with performing tuberculosis skin testing on the entire Havasupai Nation, all two or three hundred of them. I happened to be in that role because our country decided to involve itself in a war in Vietnam leading to the doctor draft for which I was a prime target. I was just finishing my medical residency at Johns Hopkins and had every inclination to avoid any activity remotely related to a Southeast Asian war that I considered of dubious roots. That was a much more dangerous direction than that for which I thought I had prepared myself, and much more dangerous than I was willing to accept without a vigorous exploration of the alternatives.

The alternative I lit upon was the Ecological Investigations Program, a CDC-run activity headquartered in Phoenix with close ties to the IHS. During my two year stint as a bona fide member of the U.S. Public Health Service, I: investigated an outbreak of dengue fever in Puerto Rico (where on an outmoded black and white TV in a B grade hotel lobby I watched the moon landing—*One Giant Step*); spent several evenings observing high-rolling gamblers doing their thing in the Puerto Rican casinos while availing myself of the free drinks; singlehandedly took on the Cocopah Reservation Shaman in an effort to suss out the path of a cluster of amoebiasis cases in a population with free access across the U.S.-Mexican border; regularly accompanied some public health nurses in their surveillance of diarrheal disease in the White Mountain Apache; enlisted the aid of the body builder, Mr. Arizona, at the local gym in toning up my medical residency-ravaged physique; and among other things, skin-tested the entire Havasupai Nation. All this while living in a tony condo in Scottsdale and compensated by your federal government. You'll have to decide for yourself whether you think that was worth your money, but I emerged alive and went on to what I like to think was a career in academic medicine that contributed to the corpus of medical knowledge and hopefully struck at least a glancing blow at human disease and misery. A mortal injury in Vietnam would have nipped that course of things in the bud. I had peers who met that fate. Who knows what price the future of civilization paid for that war?

Upon finally arriving, saddlesore and near panic at the foot of the trail, our little group was greeted by Clara Watahomigie, a Havasupai nurse who was to be our host. She ran the little clinic, managing the medical needs of her tribe on site, and, when needed, arranging for their transport to the IHS hospital in Phoenix. After we unpacked the mules and moved into the clinic (there were sleeping arrangements in the back), Clara made us coffee and went over the plans for the next couple of days. She would escort me on horseback (I wasn't sure why I needed a horse, but Clara insisted) to each of the dwellings in the village (she knew everyone in the tribe personally) along with the stash of filled syringes that we had prepared. I would place the skin tests while she recorded the event beside the appropriate name in a log. We would return in three days to read the results of the skin tests, all duly recorded.

The thought, and the reason for this herculean effort, was that since this was a pretty much isolated population (except for the tourists) there would be valuable epidemiologic information about tuberculosis transmission that might have implications for public health interventions that could decrease the incidence of the disease in the tribe. So, I reluctantly seated my aching posterior on the saddle of a thankfully sedate bay mare, and Clara and I made the rounds, injecting the antigen, maintaining the log and returning three days later to read and record the results. Unfortunately, we didn't turn up anything that changed the course of things, but it was not for lack of trying.

The Havasupai, *the people of the blue green waters*, are named for the breathtaking hue of the water spilling over Supai Falls, a tourist attraction and the source of sustenance for the food crops that grew on the canyon floor and helped to feed the residents there. In addition to steeling ourselves for our return trip to the real world (and nurturing the return of our backsides to a state of being at least pain free if not healed), during our three-day respite, we hiked the trail to the falls. We stood agape before the torrent spraying across the cliff edge into the pristine blue-green pool beneath. In fact, we marveled at the whole scene—sheer canyon walls reaching to the sky, majestic boundaries of a centuries-old Native civilization sustained by a tenacious bond to place and the good fortune of abundant beautiful water to nurture life. What must it be like to spend one's life so deeply immersed in the marvels of nature? Has to do something special to a body.

The trip back up the canyon wall toward the sky was less frightening than the one down, although not especially gentler on my backside. Emerging at the top from the mouth of the canyon's womb into the deep magenta glow of an evening sun, I was impressed with the expanse of the splayed-out plateau and the blanket of high plains scrub spread open to the vastness of the Western sky. An unlikely space in which to find myself. There was so much of it. But then I was getting pretty used to unlikely.

San Francisco Seventies

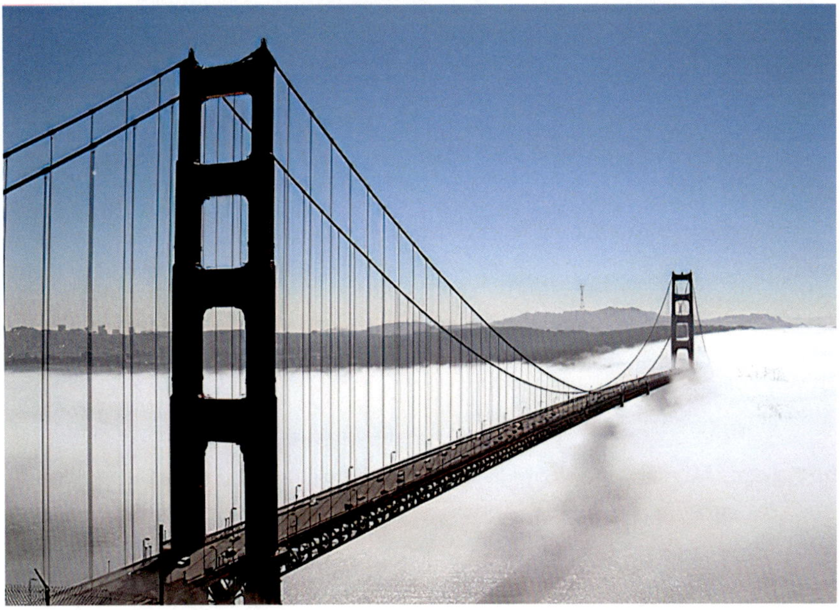

Mike Johnston/CC BY 2.0 /Wikimedia Commons

Living for a time above the clouds

Rumor has it that when physiologist and eminent teacher of human biology, Julius Comroe, rounded up his brightest colleagues in Philadelphia and convinced them to head west to the University of California San Francisco and establish the Cardiovascular Research Institute (CVRI), he soon discovered a sunroom of sorts on a high floor of Moffitt Hospital that overlooked the Golden Gate Bridge. He immediately dubbed it his *recruiting room*. At some point during a day of rigorous interviews with a faculty candidate, a time chosen when the bridge view was at its most spectacular, Dr. Comroe would escort the flagging guest to the recruiting room, present them with a cup of coffee and just leave them there alone for half an hour to contemplate their future. According to Dr. Comroe, that often did the trick. Apparently, the wily academician was not above using the beauty of the setting of the CVRI to lure promising young scholars into his fold. The strategy must have worked since the institute became a premier center for heart and lung research and the country's prime site for training the next generation of investigators and teachers in those areas.

The sight of those international orange spires of the famous bridge piercing the sky spoke of the city in the seventies—reality venturing into imagination. I arrived there in 1971. At the time the CVRI was the mecca of lung research, my chosen area of interest. For reasons mostly unrelated to the active hippie culture—the proverbial drugs, sex, and rock 'n' roll scene—I, too, was living above the clouds. Having managed to pay my dues to Uncle Sam while avoiding any direct connection with the dubious war and then landing a prime fellowship, I was moving on up.

A modest fellowship stipend and the generosity of the U.S. government's GI Bill combined to pay the rent on a small bungalow at 70 Sonora Way in Corte Madera, across the bridge in Marin County, a bit north of the much trendier (and considerably more expensive) Sausalito. So each day I crossed the Golden Gate to and from a peak educational experience on the UCSF campus perched haughtily high on Parnassus Avenue, often literally above the clouds.

The CVRI was a heady place, professional home to many whose work was widely known and admired. A day's work involved a mesmerizing drive through southern Marin County, across the iconic bridge, ending up on Mount Parnassus spending the day in the company of academic giants. After a long day in the laboratory, there was the drive back up to Marin County, time to reflect on the process of discovery that so captivated me while marveling at the beauty of the place where it happened. I was high as a kite on the whole experience. Who needed drugs?

For two years, I shared space in a small laboratory in Health Sciences East, an uncreatively named new research building, with two surgeons who had academic inclinations. Our mentor was Norman Staub, a PhD physiologist who had migrated West with Dr.

Comroe from Philadelphia. Norman, an intellect who was fixated on the scientific details of experiments, was an absolute stickler for clarity and truth in scientific writing. He had a raucous sense of humor that he was not shy to express, and loved opera. All in all, he was an interesting creature composed of many parts who was long on often devastating but usually constructive criticism of his fellows. I learned over those two years how to do rigorous research and how to communicate the results effectively to my peers and others, the basic skills that saw me successfully through the next several decades.

Of course, it was San Francisco in the early seventies, a grand sociocultural experiment fed by the cresting energies of many a youth from across the country that was lavishly spent in random efforts to discover themselves and a place where they belonged. Hard to totally ignore that. Jane Fonda (Hanoi Jane) held a rally one lunchtime on the UCSF campus and we escaped the lab to attend the spectacle. The first and only time I saw the musical *Hair* was there. Because it seemed the thing to do, I had my only brief experience with marijuana at a peer's home way up on a hill in the shadow of Mount Tamalpais on a brilliant weekend afternoon. I didn't like it. Preferred a nice, chilled, lightly herbal gin or a peaty single malt.

And Heather was born there into the midst of my life above the clouds and the grand social experiment that was the city then. Whether she osmosed enough of that ambience through her permeable neonatal skin to serve as a leg-up for her trip to becoming the remarkable woman that she is, I don't know. Maybe. Strange things sometimes happened in the City by the Bay in those odd times.

Happenstances

Shaking it for the Paying Customers

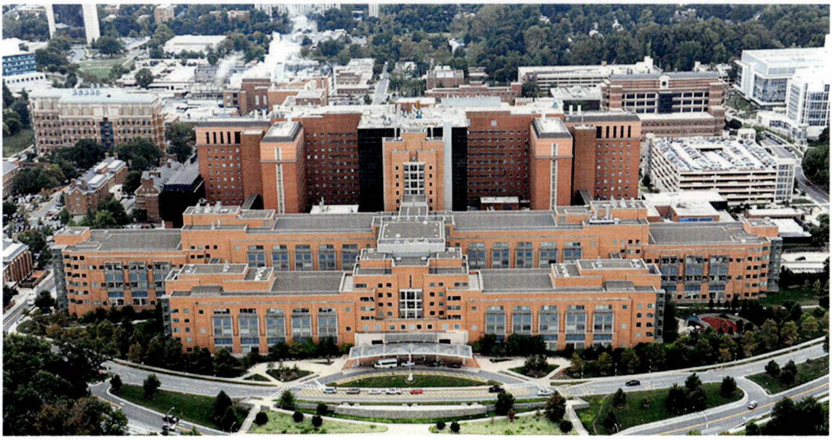

NIH: The Mother Church

Strewn confidently about a massive campus in Bethesda, Maryland, The National Institutes of Health, Mother Church of biomedical research in America, presides over a national network that connects investigators on the Bethesda campus with their compatriots in our country's other academic institutions to form the world's premier enterprise devoted to medical discovery. If you want to play in that game, you need to impress the scientists, bureaucrats, and their consultants who run the Mother Church. They pay most of the bills.

Since at least my college days, I have been impressed with the excessive value of first impressions. I would work very hard during the first semester of a course to establish myself as an "A" student. That accomplished, I tended to get the benefit of any future doubts about my performance—after all, the instructor knew that I was an "A" student—and I could ease off on the books a bit for the rest of the course.

In our interactions with fellow humans, opinions about each other are often made from woefully inadequate information—a single star turn, a fortuitous convergence of limited knowledge with an arcane problem that happens to be solved. Reputations are often made from isolated incidents that are taken as more indicative of one's potential than may be the case. Even the sophistication of a couple dozen of the country's leading scientists charged with sizing up an ambitious, young, aspiring medical investigator was no protection from what seems to be a universal human tendency.

Of course, it happened accidentally. I was barely reoriented after the long trip from San Francisco back to join the faculty at Vanderbilt and was surely too young and unproven to be running an NIH site visit that would determine the fate of a grandiose application for a Specialized Center for Lung Research (SCOR), a program requesting millions of dollars from the federal government.

An NIH site visit was something of a ritual at the time, reserved for the review of large multi-project, multi-investigator applications. A group of expert consultants was assembled who trekked with some NIH representatives to the applying institution. The principal investigator (PI) of the grant request was responsible for staging a day or two review of the content and personnel being evaluated by the expert visitors in excruciating detail. I was PI for this occasion because the program was targeted on the lung and I was the only one at Vanderbilt who was focused in that area at the time, and because I somehow summoned the audacity to convince a number of investigators, accomplished in other fields, to contrive an interest in and design a project related to the target organ. Apparently, the very large carrot of a new source of research funds outshone any suspicions of my naivete in the competitive world of the Mother Church.

The document to be reviewed was upwards of five hundred pages long. This was before word processors. I had handwritten most of the document on yellow legal pads using a calligraphy pen just to amuse myself. It was then typed by a secretary whose skills often needed to be supplemented with generous amounts of white-out; the figures, painstakingly hand drawn by artists in the medical illustrations department, were inserted; and the whole thing was copied and assembled into the tome that was distributed well in advance of the site visit to each of the participants.

The group—Vanderbilt faculty, visiting experts, NIH representatives, and various support staff—was assembled in a crowded conference room, and we were deep into the review which consisted mainly of a Q and A by the visitors, many of the Qs directed at me. Suddenly and quite unpredictably, an anecdote was transformed into a myth that affected my reputation for decades to come.

The proceedings had gone well enough until one of the reviewers caught the attention of the group by asking what sounded like a particularly difficult question. I happened to remember a graph of preliminary data that directly answered her query.

"If you will turn to the graph on page 256, I think you will find your answer," I said, thumbing through half of the document in front of me to locate the page I was referring to.

The entire group simultaneously rustled through their documents to page 256. There was a long period of silence. Some of the experts smiled.

One asked through a broad grin, "Did you memorize this entire tome, Dr. Brigham?"

Perhaps more than a little arrogantly, I assumed a serious expression, locked eyes with the questioner and replied: "I am familiar with the document."

For a long time the often-embellished story was sometimes told when my name happened to crop up in conversations about the history of lung research. I am amazed at the durability of myths among people whose profession depends so desperately on truth.

There are other examples of an unjustified bravado that landed me in circumstances where I would not otherwise have found myself. Sometimes I was graciously rescued from my overreach by older and wiser heads. My recruitment to the Vanderbilt faculty when I ended my fellowship in San Francisco is an example.

Grant Liddle, a granite-jawed Mormon who wore a hearing aid and spoke in short sentences only when he had something worthwhile to say, was probably the preeminent academic endocrinologist in the world in 1973. He chaired the department of medicine at Vanderbilt, and as a result, that institution was a global center for discovery of the detailed mechanisms of function and dysfunction of the adrenal glands and a center for training the next generation of endocrinology inclined investigators. Dr. Liddle was an intimidating presence who demanded the same excellence of those around him that he demanded of himself. His approach to recruiting faculty reflected the characteristics of his personality—gravity, commitment to excellence, a bare minimum of verbal communication, and frugality beyond what I expected even in a notoriously underpaid academic position.

The recruiting dance involved fewer phone calls and exchanges of letters than I expected. Other interested institutions were more aggressive recruiters. But Dr. Liddle was not inclined to long and complicated courtships. He quickly sized up the situation, probably sensing that I had an abiding affection for his institution, and asked, "Okay, Ken, what would it take to get you to accept the best academic offer you are likely to get?"

"Two things," I answered. "I want the title of Director of Lung Research, and I want my appointment to be associate professor of medicine with tenure."

The title was easy since I would be the only one there focused on lung research, but there was virtually no precedent for appointing a faculty candidate just finishing a fellowship at the level I brazenly requested.

A few days later, I received a terse telegram from Dr. Liddle that read, “Will recommend. Welcome to Vanderbilt.”

I was elated and immediately began to make plans to return to Nashville to launch the exciting and productive career that I anticipated.

As I am certain Dr. Liddle knew when he sent the decisive telegram, there was many a slip twixt a cup of recommendation and a lip of accomplished fact. However, I hadn’t tumbled to the message between the two short telegraphic lines. I was settled into my new laboratory in Nashville and well on my way to launching my research program when I learned that my appointment would be as assistant professor, the typical untenured starting position for new faculty fresh out of training. When I summoned up enough courage to confront my new chairman with what I considered a serious betrayal of his recruiting promise, he insisted that he had indeed recommended as I asked but that the various committees who had to approve these things would not go along. Whether that is true or not, I still don’t know, but I was stuck there whether or not I liked the process and the terms and I was wiser in the ways of how my chosen profession operated. I didn’t forget the lesson.

There are times when a well-crafted bait and switch serves the interest of everyone involved. Dr. Liddle could easily have dismissed me as an overambitious, arrogant, egotistical upstart who wasn’t worth the trouble. But he recognized naivete for what it was and did what he had to do to give me the chance of my lifetime. Dr. Liddle died after a prolonged illness during my time on the Vanderbilt faculty. I was sad. He was a great man who did well by me.

The Roar of the Greasepaint the Smell of the Crowd

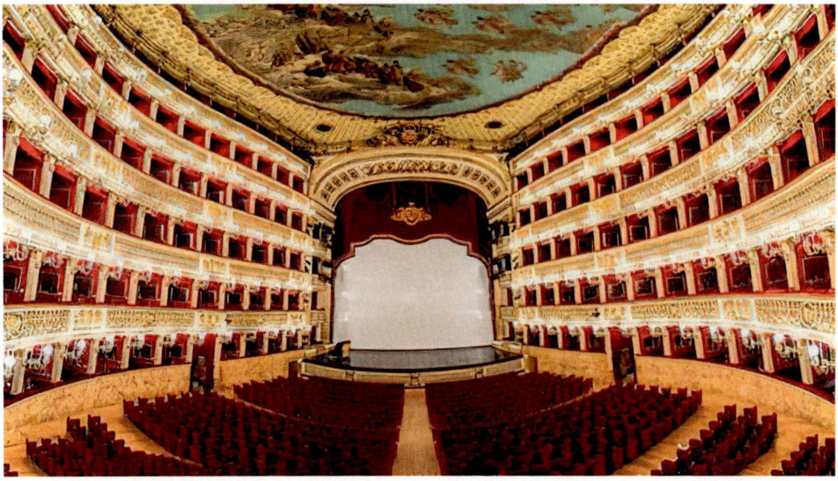

harry/Alamy Stock Photo

The fourth wall

Slouching toward the spotlight.

People with kindred interests tend to coalesce and the tendency is as strong in scientists as in anyone else. Even for us introverts (the majority, I think,) an irresistible attraction radiating from a nebulous center of recognition and power drags us toward it like a magnet pulls at scattered iron filings in a high school physics lab. We just can't help ourselves.

When groups of people congregate, they need structure—designated leaders, figureheads, spokespersons. And choosing leaders is a tricky business, especially in organizations whose members are used to democracies. It's usually done by popular vote, and if the group is large, most of the voters are pretty much flying blind with only superficial information about their choices. Since these are academics and measurable productivity—publications, grant dollars, awards, positions of power and influence in important organizations, visibility—is the currency of their profession, most voters, if they vote at all, just tally up the various accounts and cast their ballot for the top earner. The results are spotty at best.

The results are bound to be spotty because the tally of a person's academic chits has precious little to do with their ability to lead an organization. Whether the big academic earner turns out to be competent in such a role is a crapshoot, a totally random outcome of a flawed process. Might as well draw straws. But we keep doing it anyway, betting on the horse that may win when the sun shines but always loses in the rain, without first checking the weather forecast.

A surprising number of elected leaders are in painful touch with the irony of their position. You just wake up one bright morning comfortable with the prospects of spending another day going about your usual business, and you are suddenly thunderstruck with the reality that you have been thrust by the random actions of your peers into a place where you don't belong. "If they only knew who I really am," you keep repeating to yourself, "they would realize what a mistake they've made." IMPOSTER! in neon-red capital letters keeps flashing across the blank space at the edge of your mind, blinking off and on like Christmas lights.

Maybe you always felt like that, at least since you were tempted early on to drink too deeply of that toxic concoction that we call success, but you found ways to keep the feeling far enough at bay that you could function. Now you've been forced to center stage. Standing there stripped of your carefully tended façade in the searching beam of the klieg lights, the penetrating gazes of a thousand eyes are bound to see the reality: IMPOSTER!

More people than you think who live in constant full view of others feel that way—somewhat embarrassed by it all but somehow compelled to expose themselves. Some are undone by the effort. Were it not for troubled entertainers, the Hollywood psychiatric industry would fall on hard times. And there is suicide, and drugs, and other aberrant behaviors that crop up not infrequently. One's psyche can only stand so much conflict before resorting to misbehavior. So when you find yourself unexpectedly elected to lead a scientific organization, a center stage position that you are convinced you do not deserve and probably cannot do very well, where is there to hide?

I suggest that you embrace the reality of the thespians' *fourth wall*, that enigmatic barrier at the stage front that separates the actors from the audience, and do everything within your power to shore it up. Although to actors that would be a contrarian view—their profession rests on penetrating the wall, breaking through to confront face-on the dazed onlookers out there gazing through the darkness at the spectacle being staged. But for one unschooled in that profession and mainly interested in doing well enough to escape the profound embarrassment of a poor performance, there can be protected space behind the fourth wall where the private dance with recognition can be acted out while avoiding the spectacle that the reality out there threatens to lay bare.

I'm sure at least a third of the fifteen thousand members of the American Thoracic Society (ATS) sat attentively in the grand ballroom of a multi-star Boston hotel in the spring of 1990 when I hid in plain sight behind the fourth wall and stumbled through a brief welcome to the society's annual international meeting. The presidency of that organization was the only elective office that I had ever held. I was never class president, council representative, or any of those other honors conferred by classmates on their most popular fellow students. I made a half-hearted try for president of my college freshman class, encouraged by a dorm neighbor who spent most of his time pondering the breathy plaint wafting day and night from his impressive collection of Julie London records and no doubt nurturing his adolescent fantasies. It was an anemic campaign destined to fail. I reluctantly agreed to be a candidate for ATS president for the 1989-90 year feeling certain that, like my only other attempt at elected office, it was a futile exercise. But there I stood, firmly anchored behind the fourth wall, trying hard to manage the thrumming pulse of a pounding heart, and barely managing to utter a few welcoming sentences to an audience of thousands of my professional peers. I didn't feel a lot like dancing. But I headed the show for a while from my safe space behind the wall. There was room to dance had I been at ease enough to feel the beat.

There were many times in venues around the world when I felt the need to retreat to that safe space. The world of biomedical science is full of gracious people who reach out to their peers for support—information, criticism, even camaraderie. I learned from their grace and did my best to respond in kind. But I was never very good at the camaraderie thing.

Millie's Party

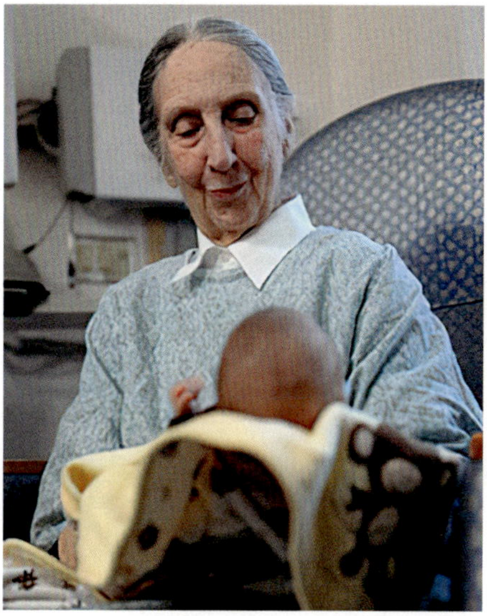

Joe Howell/Vanderbilt University Medical Center

Dr. Mildred Stahlman at work

Her given name was Mildred, but she was Millie to most of her acquaintances. My first impression of her was that of an academic giant scrunched uncomfortably into a body that stood little more than five feet tall. She was a spring-tight-wound dynamo who sometimes struggled to balance her daunting intellect with a frightening emotional irrationality that frequently threatened to erupt. I was often nervous in her presence. She could be unpredictable.

The reputation of Mildred Stahlman, MD as a pioneer in neonatology was global. Aspiring young neonatologists from everywhere flocked to Nashville for the privilege of spending some time with her at the crib side of tiny humans whose grasp on their newly conferred life was weak and often fading. Dr. Stahlman saved a lot of those fragile lives. She saved them with a savage commitment to science. I am sure there was a reservoir of love for new life behind the bloody hands that threaded those long skinny tubes through the newborns' umbilical blood vessels, slipping the catheters deftly into the heart where things were measured that defined how physiology had gone awry and tracked her efforts to put things right. Maybe there was some of a soft kind of love like a mother's gentle embrace; there were occasional hints of that. But what really drove her was a love of the realities of human biology and the skills that made it possible to manipulate the realities to sustain those tiny lives.

Millie didn't have to work that hard. Daughter of a prominent (and very rich; her father endowed five chairs at the university) citizen of the city, she could easily have relaxed her way through life, nourishing herself on the lush contents of the silver spoon that was her birthright. But she didn't do that. Instead, she took on an educational system that did not favor her gender and became one of the very few (at the time) female graduates of Vanderbilt School of Medicine. She did not choose an easy path, but she relished it. In the process of securing her medical credentials, she became enamored of the science of human physiology. She joined the Vanderbilt medical faculty and spent her life challenging scientific ignorance and introducing ailing newborn humans to the healing miracles of discovery.

"We save the lives of babies no bigger than that," Millie said with conviction as she retrieved a packaged pound of butter from her purse and plopped it with a flourish on the table before then Senator Al Gore, a few of his aides, and me.

Both Millie and I were Principal Investigators on SCOR (Specialized Centers of Research) grants from the NIH and somehow managed an audience with Senator Gore at the U.S. Capitol in Washington to lobby for continuing government support for this category of grants. The funding mechanism had its detractors even among medical researchers. SCOR grants defined the research areas that would be eligible, and many scientific traditionalists resented having the government define what research it would support. They favored *investigator-initiated* research that was an exclusive product of the creative minds of scientists and feared that dollars were being siphoned away from such projects by these politically motivated goal directed programs. Both Millie and I believed that the SCOR mechanism had attracted new research dollars and we had benefited from that. The senator from Tennessee was an effective supporter of medical science so we were in friendly territory with him, but there was a feeling that a face-on exposure to the passions of his constituents on the subject couldn't do any harm. So there we were, preaching fervently to the choir.

I was as surprised as the senator at the pound of butter thing. That was pure Millie. She was not above theater if there was a chance it would be effective, and her theatrical side seemed to be exaggerated by the heady atmosphere in the Capitol's halls that shuddered with the tremors of political power. The pound of butter story gained some notoriety for a while. Whether it had any effect on the funding of medical research is impossible to know. But I thought it made interesting theater.

Sometime around five o'clock on New Year's Eve—every New Year's Eve—several young neonatologists and their significant others bundled themselves into their cars and set about trying to locate an address on Beech Creek Road, an unpaved track that wound through the bowels of Williamson County, south of Nashville. They were French, Scottish, Swedish doctors (there were always Swedes) who were drawn to fellowships at Vanderbilt by the intellectual and personal magnet that was Dr. Stahlman. They had been invited by their mentor to spend the afternoon and evening at her home, a vintage cabin that I think had been transported log by log from its original home in Hickman County and reassembled at Millie's chosen site in a remote part of the county south of town that was not too long a commute to her job at the university. Why she chose a log cabin (she could have had any kind of abode that she wanted) and why such a difficult location (she would have been welcomed into the bosom of those of wealth and provenance in the heart of Belle Meade or anywhere else in town) were questions the answers to which were probably known only to the *Grand Dame* of neonatology herself.

Having managed to navigate the backwoods of Williamson County with sufficient skill to arrive at Millie's place, the fellows and their spouses were herded into the woods at the back of the house where there was a ritual firing of a canon that, according to legend, had been retrieved from Millie's father's yacht, and the shooting of mistletoe from the tops of trees using a rifle the origin of which I never knew. I don't think anyone was ever injured in the ritual which is surprising since I can't imagine that anyone there knew anything about firing a cannon, and the proffered rifle must have been ancient and little used.

Although Millie's party included the fellows and their spouses, they were peripheral to main action. This was one of the more exclusive New Year's affairs in the city, certainly in the university community. This was where the in-crowd reinforced their connections and new networks began to take shape—serious intent dressed up in party clothes.

As the dark and cold descended on rural Tennessee, the guests gradually trickled in. There were a few regulars—the novelist Madison Smartt Bell usually made an annual trek from Baltimore. He was the product of the union of a county judge and a lifelong friend of Millie's and had grown up not far from where the Stahlman cabin nestled into the wooded countryside. The log house seemed to be familiar territory to Mr. Bell. The current chancellor of the university was a regular, always arriving late and tuxedo-clad, giving the deliberate impression that this was only one of many such affairs that would occupy his (they were all men) evening. Millie's sisters were always present, usually settled demurely into an inconspicuous corner. This was Millie's party, not theirs. But they wouldn't miss it for the world.

To be invited to this affair was no small thing. I am sure that Millie pondered the host of possible invitees with something approaching the solemnity due a royal guest list. As one of the chosen invitees, you received the imprimatur of the *Grand Dame* and thus the implied credential as one of the local academic elite. So it was always an interesting and pretty heterogenous group—arrogant up-and-comers, proven professionals relaxing confidently at the pinnacle of their careers, high level medical school administrators (deans, deanlets, etc.), a smattering of geezers who were there mainly by dint of their tenacity, and some folks that, for obscure reasons, just happened to strike Millie's fancy. Mostly interesting people. And at least three dogs (sometimes more), refugees from the local humane society who had unfettered run of the place and took full advantage of their privilege. (The dogs slept with Millie, and she was said to judge the intensity of the winter cold by how many dogs it took to keep her warm. Apparently a three- dog night was especially chilly.)

As the consequences of consumption of the generously supplied wine and champagne took hold, conversations gained volume and intensity. Interesting conversations, not all amiable. That's what happens in a crowd of university folks. Strong minds, boundless confidence, compulsions to play to the audience, and often extreme opinions, sometimes clash in repartee that is less than friendly. Millie no doubt had an eye for such encounters when she chose the guests. She grew up in a staunch Republican household and must have been familiar with the hostility between conservatives and the traditionally liberal university crowd that spilled over from politics into almost any subject that arose. She probably relished it.

As the evening wore on and the collective energy of the group waned, an elaborate buffet appeared on the long wooden dining table. Unpretentious elegance. Traditional Southern home cooking served from what must have been Stahlman heirloom china. Genuine silver utensils. Freshly laundered and ironed linen napkins. All the trappings of dinners that must have graced the Stahlman household during Millie's youth, but food without that sort of pretense. The contrast had to be deliberate. This was Millie's party and every facet of the occasion bore her incongruous mark.

As midnight neared, the lights were dimmed and candles that decorated the Christmas tree were lit under the careful watch of Bob Cotton, Millie's trusted colleague and friend, who manned the fire extinguisher just in case. Millie took her place beside the tree. Her face illuminated by the flickering candlelight, she was a mystical visage of the promise of new time. At the stroke of midnight, she led the group in Christmas songs—carols, yes ("Adeste Fidelis," the Latin version) but secular songs, too. There was "Jingle Bells" and the perennial ode to figgy pudding ignoring the fact that Christmas Day had long since come and gone. Finally, the benediction, the strains of "Auld Lang Syne" wafting out into the frigid night to the rhythm of the ponderous trudge of Father Time.

There was a post-climactic breakfast of mushy black-eyed peas and cured country ham almost too salty for human consumption—gestures to the Southern folk myth that black-eyed peas eaten on New Year's Day assured a profitable year to come. As best I could tell, most people took token portions of the food. The party was over and most of the guests were looking for ways to leave with the grace that Millie and her party deserved.

I must have attended a couple dozen of these affairs over my thirty-odd year career on the university faculty. I very much appreciated the invitations, but I never felt as though I belonged there. These were people I valued and respected, but they were by and large not my kind. "IMPOSTER!" often intruded on my thoughts of the evening.

Two Miracles

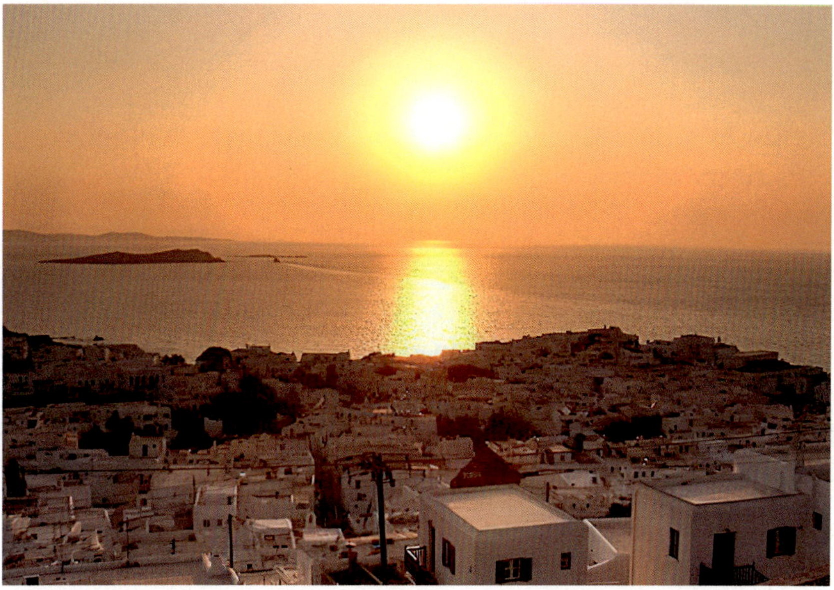

dronepicr/CC BY 2.0/Wikimedia Commons

A miracle

On the Greek island of Mykonos, there is a long pier that juts for a hundred yards or so westward from the shore. Heather and I walked out to the end of it just as the sun was setting on a balmy evening and watched the emerald sea swallow its solar prey down to the last red crescent that seemed reluctant to yield its view of *terra firma* before finally taking the plunge, giving over the duties of illumination to a brilliant yellow moon, just rising from behind where we sat. We did not speak.

I believe that our universe probably started with the big bang and happened according to knowable laws of physics. I also am aware that the glory of the sunset that my daughter and I watched that balmy evening in Greece was, as sunsets always are, a consequence of atmospheric conditions, the rotation of the planets, and their positions relative to each other in space, perfectly predictable phenomena. I don't need to postulate a mystical force that goes about its business without regard for the laws that govern the behavior of matter. Reality is perfectly fine with me as a consequence of things (and people for that matter) behaving in ways that are either entirely predictable from equations that someone could write or will be able to write once some more of the science is worked out. I don't need the *deus ex machina* explanation—then a miracle happened—for how the universe works.

Does that mean that I don't believe in miracles? Not really. Maybe it depends on what you call a miracle. I would claim, even more than thirty years hence, that watching the sunset that evening in Mykonos with Heather, my daughter who was just blossoming into the beautiful woman whom she subsequently became, had all the elements I need to proclaim it a miraculous experience. I guess that means that I define miracles as feelings rather than events. On that miraculous evening in Greece, nobody was raised from the dead; no water was turned into wine; no demons were cast out; no leper was made whole again; no one ascended into the heavens. The brilliant evening sun just gently sank from the western sky into the sea, a nightly spectacle as predictable as the rising of the moon or the morning reappearance of the sun emerging in the eastern sky in all its fiery brilliance refreshed from its evening respite in the seabed. But Heather and I were there to *feel* it happen.

And, I confess, her existence was much of the substance of the miracle for me. She, the incarnation of the very human capacity (and urge) to procreate, was miracle number one. I am sure that, once our species is sufficiently enlightened, what I felt as I watched my only child emerge, bloody and squawking, into a world that would be a better place for her having lived in, will be better understood. But I had no need to understand what happened to me early on that summer day in 1973 in San Francisco. I still do not need an objective explanation. None of the belabored clichés do the trick. In an instant, I was bound forever to a new inhabitant of our planet with an intensity that I had not anticipated and continue to relish after almost half a century. It is not a feeling that wanes with time. "Love never fails," Saint Paul informed the Christians at Corinth. While I am not sure about everything that the apostle wrote and believed, he got this right. Time and life have nurtured the bond that emerged quite suddenly early on a June morning in that city that has its own take on magic.

I reflected on the miracle that happened all those years ago as Heather and I felt the sunset from our vantage point on Mykonos. There seems to be a synergy among miracles.

A Time to Die

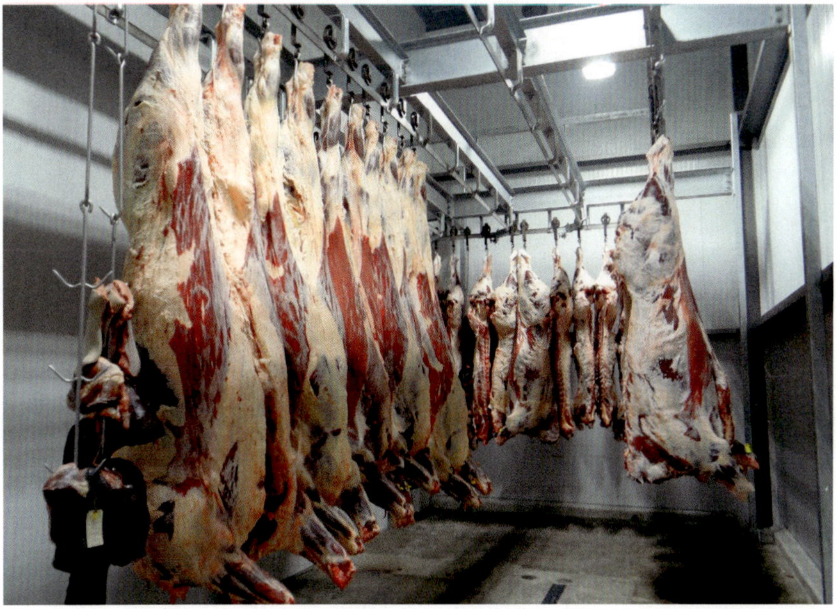

blackriv/Pixabay

The killing floor

The on-site supervisor of the slaughterhouse, a white single story block building sitting in the middle of what had been a farm just outside the Nashville city limits, was nice enough on the phone.

"Sure," he said. "Come on out. We'll do what we can to accommodate you, but you'll need to stay out of our way. And it's not a pretty site, the killing floor. You'll need to forget about the niceties of the university. This place ain't no ivory tower. We're about the business of slaughtering animals and we don't worry very much about appearances. We just get the job done so you can have your beefsteak when you want it." He may have chuckled to himself; I couldn't be sure.

The call and the subsequent forays to the slaughterhouse were a result of a notion by one of our pathologists with a special interest in how the cells lining blood vessels (endothelial cells) interacted with cells circulating in the blood to either maintain healthy vessels or to initiate disease. For some reason, she thought that bovine tissue and cells were likely to be a good model of what happened in humans. Realizing that a lot of cows were killed for food, we wondered whether we could prevail upon the slaughterers to let us collect small amounts of blood and lung blood vessels for study in the laboratory. Although I was not above killing animals if the likely benefit to humans justified it, if we could achieve the same result without having to decide whether that was the case—dodging the bigger "time to die" question—this approach might be both a tactical and a moral winner.

That bigger question is a real gut wringer. Clearly all life is transient so that there is a time when each living creature will die one way or another. But a *time to die*, that is, a specific time for life to end for each one of earth's creatures? Hard to tell from what we can know. However, the pervading truth of the slaughterhouse—arrive alive and leave as parcels of dead meat—was happening anyway. Perhaps we could even lend some dignity to the situation.

There is no dignity to be had on the killing floor. There is something transcendently ugly about deliberate death that defies any efforts to nice it up. The people doing it do not appear to need a prevailing philosophy to rationalize what they do. It is a job and they are about it. From the paralyzing thud of the bolt gun that is the beasts' entrée onto the clanking apparatus that strings them up and moves them methodically, head dangling, to the final exit of the carcass to the cold room, the killing floor is a concatenation of sensations that brook no diversion from the goal. Knives flash, sprays of blood bathe the place, and the marshalled battalion of gradually dismantled bovine remains steadily clanks its way toward the cold to rest the carcasses a while before they are subjected to the culinary skills of their higher order brethren and eventually to the digestive systems of those of their killers and their like who can afford the tab.

I had the distinct and very immediate feeling that I risked my life on each of the visits we made to the slaughterhouse. While my colleague dissected some tissue from the removed lungs on a stainless steel bench, my job was to scale a blood-soaked and very slippery steel ladder to a small perch beside the passing line of bovine carcasses carrying a one hundred cc syringe with a very large needle. As the bodies passed by, I was to stick the carotid artery and withdraw as much blood as I could in the time available. The disassembly line did not slow for me and I don't think anyone was especially interested in how insecure I felt. The workers may even have been amused to have a university professor as captive in their netherworld where I was unsure of myself and they were in charge. There is something about competence and power.

My pathologist colleague and I would leave the place after each visit clutching our prized specimens to our bloodied shirtfronts. I privately hoped that the effort would fail to yield anything interesting, that I would be spared experiencing the misery and fear of the unseen world that underlay the appetite of Americans for beef. But that didn't happen for a while.

A time to die. As I pondered that dictum, the killing floor kept coming to mind. Medicine is preoccupied with death. The first person I watched die was my father when I was fifteen and he was suffering the end stages of metastatic prostate cancer. Even at the time, I thought that it was too late for him to die. He had wasted away, body and soul. He had clung to an imitation of life that no longer brought joy to him or those who cared for him. If he had a prescribed time to die, he overshot the goal. I have since watched many people die. If the timing of their final breath had something to do with the grand cosmic plan, it wasn't apparent to me. I thought most of the people I watched die were doing it too soon or too late. In dealing with life's really big issues, like death, timing is a tricky business to predict. It's too easy to miss the target even if you know what you're aiming at.

So don't send me back to the slaughterhouse. I've been there and done that and feel no need to repeat the experience. It is sufficient to my understanding of life and death to know that there is a killing floor, a netherworld where animals are systematically killed and disassembled to meet the desires of our society. And it is enough to make me wonder about whether there is a time to die but that we aren't clever enough to understand or to deal with the concept.

Old Overcoat

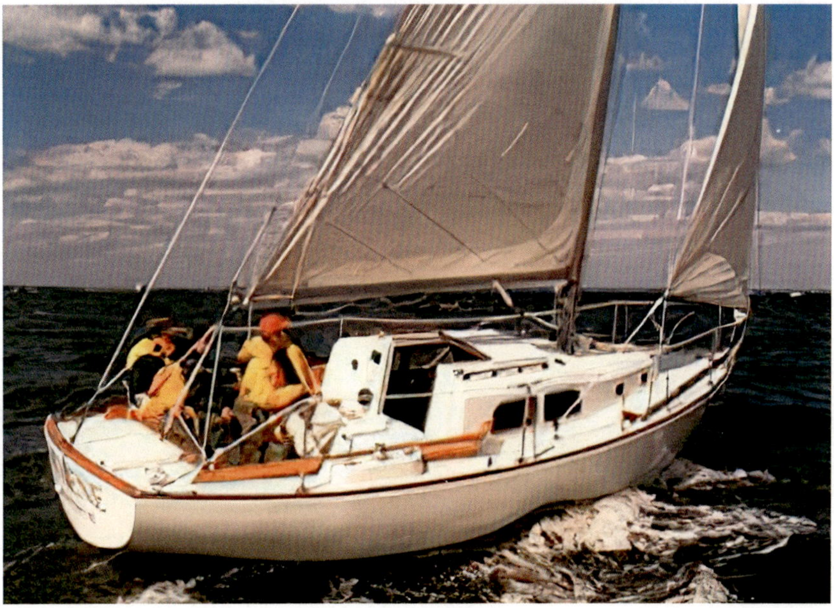

Pearson Renegade

Over the bounding main

Bo Sheller introduced me to rye whiskey, specifically to Old Overholt, the oldest continually maintained whiskey made in America. He also introduced me to the thrill of maneuvering a twenty-seven-foot sloop about the far reaches of Old Hickory Lake on days when we yielded to the elemental call of a brisk wind, deserted other obligations, and headed for the water. Not infrequently, those two indulgences coincided. I suppose such things happen when you're of a mind to indulge.

Old Overcoat, we renamed the whiskey; Bo was fond of toying with words. Maybe he developed that habit early (he was the son of Louisiana schoolteachers). Or maybe it was a result of his university education—The University of the South (Sewanee) English major and protégé of the Agrarian author, Andrew Lytle, one of that institution's better-known writers. Or perhaps it was a British thing absorbed during his years at Oxford as a Rhodes scholar. Hard to tell how his many influences melded into the man I came to know about as well as he permitted that of anyone.

Although I had grown up essentially landlocked, I had always been intrigued by sailing. I think the attraction was the essential challenge of managing the interaction of the sails with the wind to keep things moving in the right direction. Well, that and the language. Nautical jargon ("naughty-cal," Bo called it, as in "I love it when you talk naughty-cal") was irresistible, a vast storehouse of metaphors gift-wrapped in the lilting rhythms of the sea. What more could a lover of words ask of the language gods?

When I bought my first sailboat (a small Catalina sloop), I'd had no experience sailing. I read books on the topic, including nautical dictionaries, and made serious efforts to follow the instruction in the books with mixed results. However, I was hooked. From the Catalina, I moved on to a shiny, new twenty-one-foot Benneteau. That was a beautiful boat, but I really wanted a wheel instead of a tiller, a silly reason for trading up that lent truth to the observation of the man who sold me the Catalina that *no one buys just one sailboat; your first one is always too small.* Well, my first one was too small and my second one didn't have a steering mechanism to my liking and so I bought number three, the used twenty-seven-foot Pearson with an inboard motor and a lovely chrome wheel on which Bo and I spent many a breezy afternoon exploring the lake while often consuming the better part of a fifth of *Old Overcoat*.

Although I was technically Bo's boss (among his numerous accomplishments, he had become James R. Sheller, MD, and moved on to be chief medical resident and postdoctoral fellow at UCSF, the position from which I recruited him to Vanderbilt), I don't think the full meaning of that relationship ever totally sunk in on either of us. That was probably a good thing. It gave Bo a great deal of professional freedom to build a career with minimal interference from me, and

I had expert sailing lessons during many pleasant afternoons on the lake, not to mention a new appreciation of rye whiskey.

I didn't know of his love of and expertise at sailing until sometime after Bo was settled back in Nashville and into his new faculty position. Typical of the private young man that he was, it was some time before he mentioned his Scottish mentor in the sport that apparently consumed a large fraction of his two years at Oxford, compliments of Mr. Rhodes. That was big water sailing of the old school. Bo described being lashed to the main mast with a sextant during a storm to read the boat's position in the stars from a reasonably stable place. I couldn't imagine it.

And as you would have expected, he had mastered the language. He must have inherited the pedagogy gene from his parents. I could not have had a better teacher.

The Joy of Irrelevance

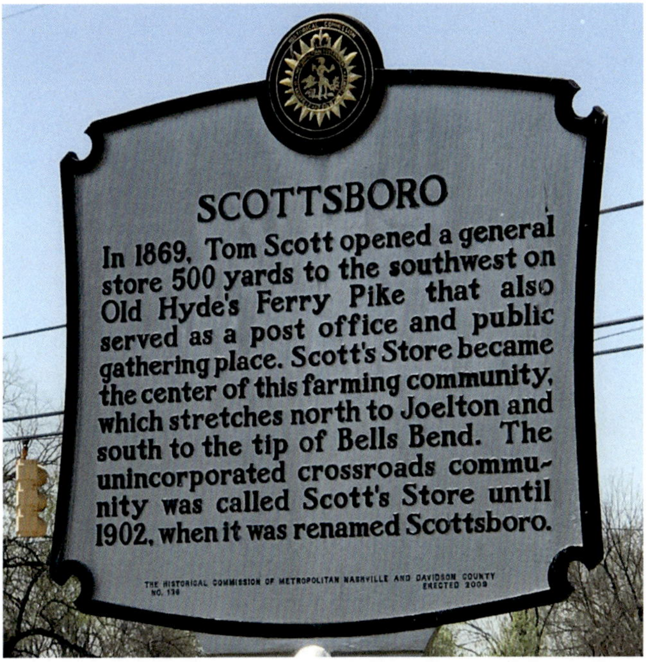
SCOTTSBORO
In 1869, Tom Scott opened a general store 500 yards to the southwest on Old Hyde's Ferry Pike that also served as a post office and public gathering place. Scott's Store became the center of this farming community, which stretches north to Joelton and south to the tip of Bells Bend. The unincorporated crossroads community was called Scott's Store until 1902, when it was renamed Scottsboro.

Duane and Tracy Marsteller/HMdb.org

Ashland City Highway at Old Hickory Blvd

Does place matter?

According to the historic marker located at the center of Scottsboro, Tennessee, a small but durable settlement a few miles north of Nashville, the single historic event related to the place that deserved mention was the establishment in 1869 of a general store by someone named Tom Scott. I spent several of my formative years living on a small farm two miles from that site and have no reason to believe that the marker overlooked anything more significant in Scottsboro's history. As best I could tell, the people who lived there, even if you include the area from Joelton to the far end of Bells Bend (I suppose that would be the Scottsboro metropolitan area), spent most of their time and energy doing what they had to do to make a living for themselves and their families. Probably not much time left for doing the kind of stuff that the historic marker people would find interesting enough to include on their commemorative plaques. Nobody I knew there would have cared much about such things one way or the other.

My life in Scottsboro was difficult. Although I learned a lot about how humans manage to relate to the plant and animal world in ways that allow us to live in a complicated ecosystem, and even thrive if one is lucky, unless you start out ahead of the game (i.e., have money), that road is hard and often unforgiving. After leaving the Scottsboro farm following the death of my father and getting on with my very different life, I never missed the farm and vowed to find some way to deal with the realities of our natural ecosystem that would produce a favorable result without requiring the kind of hands-on intimacy—the blood and guts at the front lines of survival—that seemed to me necessary if you chose to live too close to the sources of life's essentials. I had no problem with hard work but wanted some liberty to choose a kind of work that suited me. I was through with Scottsboro, both the place and the metaphor. At least I thought so.

But then I could not have anticipated that I would be invited to become a founding member of the *Scottsboro Culinary and Literary Society*. Years after I had given any significant thought to the place, I happened to sit next to Tom John, a lanky North Carolinean rheumatologist who was a fellow Vanderbilt faculty member. He was married to Brenda Butka, a multitalented pulmonologist who had joined the faculty of the division that I directed, and the occasion was our regular Friday afternoon division happy hour at a local watering hole. At some point probably well into the afternoon festivities, Tom, on the authority of and no doubt at the urging of Charlie Ray, the lawyer who conceived the proposed culinary and literary organization, duly extended the invitation along with a lengthy and not terribly coherent recitation of the proposed rules of governance. Here is what I think might have been a founding document should anyone involved have been inclined to write one:

Founding Rules of the Scottsboro Culinary and Literary Society (SCLS)

Consistent with the society's three guiding principles—eccentricity, irrelevance, and mirth—the following rules shall govern activities.

1. The founding members shall have some more or less direct connection with Scottsboro, the place. [My connection was historic, but both Charlie (and wife Sandra) Ray and Tom and Brenda had made their homes in Scottsboro, neither a thriving neighborhood of young Nashville professionals nor a suburb in the throes of gentrification, but appropriate to the personalities and proclivities of the people involved.] See guiding principle *eccentricity*.

2. The group shall meet at irregular intervals to be determined by an unspecified random process rotating among the homes of the founding members, in sequence unless there are exceptions.

3. The hosts for each meeting shall be responsible for providing food and drink, preferably of a quality equal to or exceeding that to which the founding members are accustomed.

4. The hosts for each meeting shall be responsible for a program, presentation, or other intellectual activity either by themselves or by (an) invitee(s) of their choosing.

5. The chosen intellectual activity shall attempt to avoid professional or other interests of the founding members and any topic of immediate social concern. See guiding principle *irrelevance*.

6. Should any of the founding members violate these rules, the offender shall be subject without mercy to the unbridled amusement of their fellow members. See founding principle *mirth*.

7. A volunteer from among the founders shall be responsible for recording the proceedings of each meeting that shall include a menu, a description of the program, an account of the evening's discussion, and other items of interest. These documents taken together shall comprise the *Annals of the Scottsboro Culinary and Literary Society* and shall be preserved as the society's historical record.

8. In recognition of the difficulties likely to be involved, and the importance of preserving the society's guiding principles, Rule No.7 may be omitted if there is no volunteer to undertake the task or at the inclination of any meeting's host or of the founders as a group or individually.

I could see nothing in Tom's description of the proposed organization with substance enough to support the foundation and sustenance of a society of any kind and did not respond immediately. However, after another glass of wine and some brief rumination on the proposal, I realized that the point was that there was no point, and thus became drawn irresistibly to the idea. I accepted the offer on the spot, which I suppose means that the SCLS was founded in the bar of a restaurant on Division Street across the way from the campus of Vanderbilt University. Although I have not checked recently, I am quite certain that, consistent with the society's ethos (and a general lack of interest), there is no commemorative plaque there to mark the occasion.

Against all odds, the SCLS was established and lasted for well over a decade. On the occasion of the society's tenth anniversary, Charlie Ray had T-shirts made that bore a David Levine caricature of (I think) Shakespeare from the *New York Review of Books* with the caption, *A Decade of Irrelevance.* Although the society continued after that for some time, I think of Charlie's T-shirts as its obituary. Of course, a premature obituary would not have been inconsistent with the broad liberties conferred by the society's guiding principles for what it chose to do.

A couple of memorable evenings.

Amateur astronomer and cosmologist (and incidental lawyer) Mark Manner used Guy Ottewell's *The Earth as a Peppercorn* model to convert cosmic distances to earth units. Based on that model, Mark recreated our solar system by placing tokens of each of the planets at relatively correct distances from an arc of the soccer ball-sized sun imagined to occupy the southwest corner of our Printers Alley apartment and proceeding down Church Street to the southwest for two hundred paces to the pinhead-sized Pluto. The appropriately lubricated group made the trek enhanced by Mark's erudite cosmological repartee and returned to Printers Alley for the evening meal better educated if no closer to the intriguing significance of superimposing cosmic distances and sizes on our very Earth-sized Nashville neighborhood. I have no idea what any observers thought about what we were doing, but they were probably wrong and it didn't seem to matter.

Founding rules No. 5 and No. 6 were often invoked, predictably so by a group of people passionate about life in general as well as their chosen professions. What would you expect from a group that included three doctors and a lawyer among its founding members, professions that are often chosen for their commitment to the health and well-being of their fellow men? An occasion comes to mind when founder Brenda Butka and the evening's guest architect, Manuel Zeitlin, entangled themselves in an increasingly loud exchange related to the design of the local Montessori school. As the volume of the exchange grew, the initial pause in conversation by other society members broke suddenly into uproarious laughter (dictated by Rule No. 6) that with a generous replenishment of wine served to recoup the proper ambience for the occasion. There are times for venting one's passion for education and other equally important social matters, but this was not one of them.

And there was unanticipated beauty. A dinner at a small inn in Joelton (distal edge to the north of the village of Scottsboro) was followed by an invitation to the owners' basement gallery that displayed the largest collection of Inuit stone sculptures that either my wife Arlene or I had ever seen. Arlene grew up in Winnipeg and was something of an expert on Inuit art and she was spellbound by the display—ebony sculptures of all sizes and subjects sequestered in the basement of an out-of-the-way inn in Joelton, Tennessee. There was no discernible reason for its existence and no possibility that we would ever have known of it except for a group of people bent on finding irrelevance, eccentricity, and mirth among the important reasons for their residing on our planet of eternal surprise.

Does place matter?

Would something like the Scottsboro society have ever existed if the founders, like many of their peers, had put their Nashville stakes down at 4,000-square-foot McMansions in Brentwood? Although it could be plausibly argued that affluent neighborhoods like Brentwood have their own brands of irrelevance, I suspect that they carry with them more angst and sleeplessness than those of the Scottsboro folks. Granted, the Scottsboro neighbors are more preoccupied with matters of immediate concern to life's necessities than the frills of affluence, but was it the people? Was it the Scottsboroans' attitude toward life that captured the imaginations of the outlanders who founded the society? Or was it the *place*, the green hills and fertile fields that were home to those people who shared both a concern for others of their kind and the freebies that come with being human that are the raw materials for happiness and joy?

The roads that lead to a satisfying life are as many and varied as their travelers. But I suspect that place matters to them all.

To Rio on a Whim

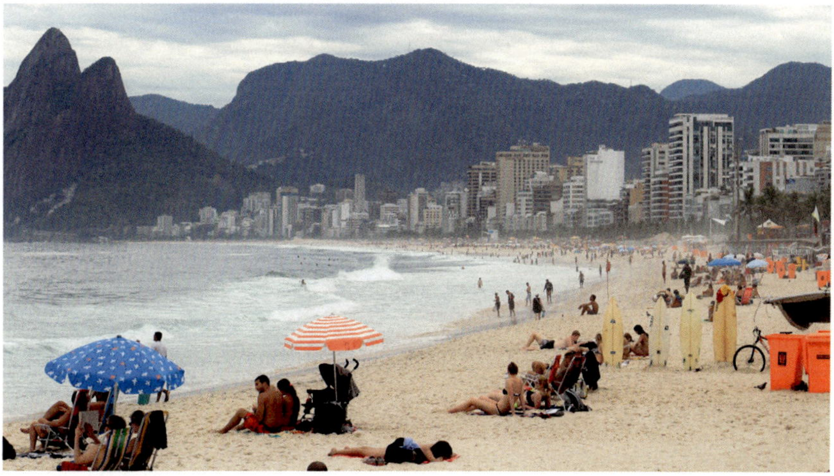

Xiuli Tan/CC0/Wikimedia Commons

Ipanema

Several hours after departing Nashville on a southbound flight path aimed at an obscure spot on the eastern border of a different continent, the well-travelled Varig aircraft bounced heavily onto the tarmac at the airport serving Montevideo, Uruguay, and taxied to an aging terminal to disgorge its half-load of weary travelers into the blinding glare and searing heat of the South American noonday sun. The flight had been long and not especially pleasant. The now defunct Varig Airlines was probably already on its last legs at the time and so was no longer paying much attention to creature comforts. Maybe it never did. Maybe the German founder of the Brazilian company weaved his spartan ethos into its soul.

The first impression of the South American city that I recall was the image of a perfectly restored 1957 Chevrolet parked in front of the college dormitory that was my assigned quarters for the duration of the meeting. In 1957, I was a senior in high school when my probably too trusting brother-in-law loaned me his spanking new Chevy for prom night. The sight of that iconic machine, chrome festooned tail fins gleaming in the sun, sitting there as good as new by the curbside in such a distant time and place was disorienting. I think that scene lent an air of unreality to the whole trip.

It was a large international meeting of scientists with special interests in diseases of the lungs and it is common for such meetings to use the facilities of their universities to house and feed their professional visitors. Trying to live like a student again may have had a romantic appeal to guests who were more familiar with multi-star hotels, but the spare realities of the student life rarely lived up to the dream. One does become accustomed to *en suite* bathrooms with plenty of hot water and twenty-four-hour room service. One feels no compelling reason to adjust to a less commodious style. After all, been there, done that. But then, I was there on my host's peso, so it was what it was. Isn't there some guiding principle about paying fiddlers and calling tunes?

I was invited to Montevideo as one item on an extensive roster of speakers, although the meeting theme was something to do with tuberculosis and my research was related to the lung but had precious little connection with TB. As it turned out, most of the audience was not fluent in English and so heard my talk through an interpreter of unknown skill. Maybe the relevance of my presentation to the meeting theme didn't really matter that much.

This was when I was near my professional peak and many of the invitations I got were based on my published work rather than any expectation of a grand performance. I was a star on paper, but not reliably so in the flesh. My name on the list of speakers was effective window dressing that had some appeal to potential paying customers and how it played out was probably not that important. I found that true of scientific meetings in general. The carefully crafted promise was elegantly marketed in relevant journals and (more recently) on professionally designed web sites, but once you scrabbled together the resources necessary to pay for travel, hotel, registration fees, etc., and arrived on the site, you usually spent most of your time in the hotel bar shooting the breeze with whomever you encountered there. Attending a scientific meeting was more a social experience than a professional one. But then we Homo sapiens are social animals.

Jim Hogg was as Canadian as it is possible to be. He might, like his brother, have joined the Royal Canadian Mounted Police (RCMP) and spent his life chasing the Canadian version of bad guys but that would have deprived the scientific world of the curiosity and insight of one of its leading lung pathologists. Jim left McGill University in Montreal for St. Paul's Hospital in Vancouver mid-career and continued to distinguish himself in the lung research community by his careful and insightful observations of lung pathology. I don't remember when we first met, but whenever it was, I felt an immediate affinity with Jim that never waned as we whiled away the years, comfortably ensconced in our different experiences of academic medicine.

Noting that we were both invited speakers to the Montevideo conference, we arranged to meet and spend some time together exploring that part of Uruguay. There was a practical reason for connecting since we were a part of an English-speaking minority among the advertised participants, but we also relished the chance to spend some time together. At least I did. It is sometimes hard to tell what a Canadian relishes.

Over several days Jim and I, map in hand, covered most of Montevideo on foot, taking in the sights and catching up on personal and professional happenings. As the time to leave for home neared, Jim suggested that we go to Rio. I still have no idea why, but it seemed like a good idea to me. I was in no hurry to escape the unreality of this whole experience and a detour with Jim through a place that neither of us had ever visited seemed an amiable way to exploit the opportunity offered by a disconnect from reality. The rest of my life would still be there after Rio. At the time it didn't seem to matter that much.

"Do you speak English?" I asked the handsome, brown-skinned young man behind the counter at the Brazilian embassy.

"No," he replied in flawless English. "Do you speak Portuguese?"

It turned out that Canadians did not need a visa to visit Brazil, but Americans did. So, Jim trudged with me to the embassy and waited patiently for me to identify the essential bureaucratic hoops, clear them—forms, photographs, etc.—and thus earn the passport stamp that was necessary to get me past the Brazilian authorities at the Rio airport and on to our Ipanema beach destination. The less than accommodating embassy clerk was a minor annoyance. Jim and I were deep into dreams of a postcard Rio beach and our fantasy would not be spoiled by a bureaucrat too clever for his job.

We spent only a couple of days in Rio. Most of one day was spent enjoying a fifth of good bourbon that someone had given to Jim and talking, the way old friends do when the opportunities are scarce. We jogged on the beach, picking our way through the crowds of sun worshippers arrayed about the broad swath of white sand separating the forest of condo towers from the ocean's contented sighs and bottomless blue promise of a world without boundaries, a seagoing world that lived by its own rules.

Alas, I eventually returned to Nashville and reconnected to my private reality. But I often dreamed of a place that was not so firmly trussed to that world.

In the Wake of an Assassin

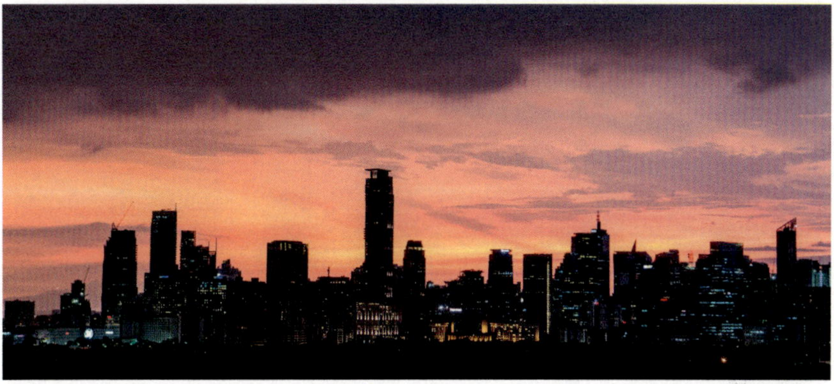

Andrey Andreyev/Unsplash

Manila at Rest

I arrived at Manila International Airport on Monday, August 22, 1983, the day after Benigno Aquino, Jr., a popular dissident senator, was assassinated, shot through the head in broad daylight probably near the same spot on the tarmac where my flight touched down. I was unaware of that event and I had no idea that the slight woman wearing a dark dress and a somber face with whom I shared the flight would three years later be the Philippine president and *Time* magazine's Woman of the Year. Corazon Aquino, the self-described plain housewife of the slain senator, was returning from exile in the U.S. She went on to seize the momentum of her husband's murder to engineer the end of the despotic Marcos regime and to bend the arc of her country's future in a new direction.

At the time, I was unaware of who the Aquinos were and of the political ferment set in motion by Benigno's murder. However, as soon as I got off the plane and entered the terminal, I knew that something of major proportions was afoot. The sprawling terminal, no doubt usually teeming with hordes of travelers on their way to distant corners of the world, was eerily vacant except for squads of uniformed young men with assault rifles slung casually over their shoulders who paced about, the sharp crack of their boots on the tile floor echoing in the emptiness. Itchy fingers caressing the triggers of their weapons, the soldiers' eyes constantly scanned the room, appearing to search for any hint of irregularity sufficient to justify using potentially lethal force in what was a very irregular scene.

I was petrified. I had never imagined being that close to the business end of a single Uzi, much less an airline terminal full of them. Although I had the proper documents to justify my presence there, this reception committee was a far cry from the drowsy, rotund customs official who usually gave a disinterested glance at one's credentials upon entering a strange country. The escort who was to meet me at the arrival gate was nowhere to be seen. I was alone, surrounded by heavily armed young men, in a very strange place, and my only advance instructions were to meet up at the airport with a representative of the organization that was hosting this visit. He would get me to a hotel and give me the rest of the information that I needed. That was Plan A. But no representative, no hotel, no information. And no Plan B.

I felt as alone as at any time in my life before or since. I dared not appear to the armed guards as though I had no purpose for being there, and so I strode determinedly in random directions for a while, trying to decide what to do. Since the airport was obviously in lockdown, there was no way for my contact to meet me at the gate or probably anywhere else in the building. If he was there at all, he must be outside, likely in front of the terminal where I would have to exit unless I decided to camp out inside until the lockdown ended and he could get to our planned rendezvous point. Who knew how long that would be? And what about the guys with guns? I concluded that hanging around waiting for something positive to happen was not a viable plan. Hoping that my Philippine contact had arrived at the same conclusion, I finally exited the terminal and found him pacing back and forth near the curb displaying a hand-crafted sign with my name on it. He looked relieved when I approached him and introduced myself.

As we drove to the hotel, my host, a middle-aged, twitchy man who purported to be some sort of mid-level government official, gave me his version of the situation—the previous day's murder of the dissident senator, the arrival of the senator's widow on the same flight that I was on, the lockdown of the airport, and his version of what was likely to happen next including the possibility of a full-blown revolution. Apparently, the natives were restless and maybe the fuse had been lit.

Although he claimed to be a representative of the government, meaning the Marcos regime, the tone of my escort's long description of the situation sounded like he had some sympathy for the Aquinos and some excitement about the possible consequences of recent events. I wondered if a real revolution was in the offing and probed a little about that, but apart from his obvious excitement, he didn't volunteer anything more. He did confirm that the touring American medicine show was to proceed as originally conceived. That made me think that the powers that be might not be taking the events of the last couple of days as seriously as they deserved. Although I knew nothing about revolutions, either for or against, if that was a possibility, I would have thought that the government should be concentrating its energies on something other than the welfare of visiting doctors who didn't have a dog in that fight. I didn't want to be there, but I was stuck, trapped by my lifelong habit of keeping promises, even when it was inconvenient. Inconvenience was one thing, but I hadn't thought about the possibility that what I considered an admirable personality trait could be dangerous. I was generally pretty practical, but I wasn't brave. The very thought of trying to negotiate a way through the crossfire of a battle that shouldn't have concerned me one way or the other, shook me to my essentially pacifist core.

Although I usually paid close attention to what I wore, I had never owned a *barong tagalog*. Apparently the current first lady, Imelda Marcos, though faced with a possible upheaval in her comfortable life resulting from the Aquino murder, found time to concern herself with the wardrobe of foreign visitors. So a young man wielding a tape measure and claiming to be a tailor sent by Ms. Marcos herself appeared at my hotel door and insisted on taking several measurements of my upper body for the purpose of creating for me a made-to-measure barong tagalog, the traditional elaborately embroidered formal Philippine shirt. That was okay with me, although completely unnecessary. I was there, ensconced in a very nice hotel, and fully informed of the plans for the visit. I was okay for the time being and wasn't sure that a barong tagalog would do much to improve my situation. However, the same young man reappeared a day later with the promised shirt, a lovely example of fine needlecraft, which I never wore. I kept it in my closet for several years, but it is no longer there, probably cast aside like so many relics of unique destinations that left no real urge to either prolong the memory or to repeat the experience. In retrospect, the first lady's gift may have been a symbol of how important trivia can become when the foundations of one's world begin to tremble.

There were four of us Americans who were invited by the Philippine government to spend a few days touring the far-flung collection of islands that make up that country and staging dog and pony shows for health care professionals at locations selected to reach as many interested Philippines as possible. The functions were held in large auditoriums that were generally jampacked. Most of the medical community there appeared to be Western-oriented, although we visitors would probably not have been exposed to the traditional folk medicine practices that presumably also thrived. The audiences were receptive, and we were royally entertained as well. The political drama that I confronted upon arrival didn't seem to bother the locals all that much. If I raised the subject in a private conversation, the response was usually to change the topic to something related to medicine, which was, after all, the reason I was there.

There was a luau in our honor on the beach in Cebu City. We were loaded up on what must have been a ripe-for-decommissioning Philippine Airlines plane for the hour and a half flight south from Manila to the oldest city in the country, center of a thriving shipping industry. The island of Cebu was one of the country's more prosperous regions and the city looked it—skyscrapers, luxury apartment blocks, and an undercurrent of bustle that suggested serious activity. We arrived in the afternoon before our performance scheduled for the next day and the evening's entertainment was an elaborate luau that would have turned a Hawaiian green with envy.

The beachfront venue was decorated with colorful streamers and Japanese paper lanterns. There was music strummed on some species of stringed instrument that didn't look familiar to me. Young girls in grass skirts danced what looked to me like a credible imitation of the hula. A long table was presided over by an actual roast pig with glazed eyes and mouthing a bright red apple. Every imaginable and many unimaginable kinds of seafood, vegetables, fruits, and native sweets crowded the table, spilling over the edges in places. Some kind of punch tasting of liberal amounts of spirits was being dispensed by barefoot, handsome young men and women circulating among the crowd.

The spectacle was a serious effort to stage an evening of novel entertainment and it was pleasant enough except for the recurring feeling that the scene was misplaced. The theme of the occasion was not authentic; nothing about it spoke of local culture. And an elaborate party for visiting Americans on a Philippine beach almost before the mutilated body of the country's leading dissident was cold, felt wrong. As the evening wore on, I felt more and more like a stranger in a strange land, a displaced person washed ashore on a tropical island whose inhabitants borrowed their culture from others and who seemed little concerned about the current and future state of their country. I would do what I had promised, but I was anxious to have the whole thing over with and to head back to more familiar territory.

I was in a wrong place.

Discovery

Soul Mates

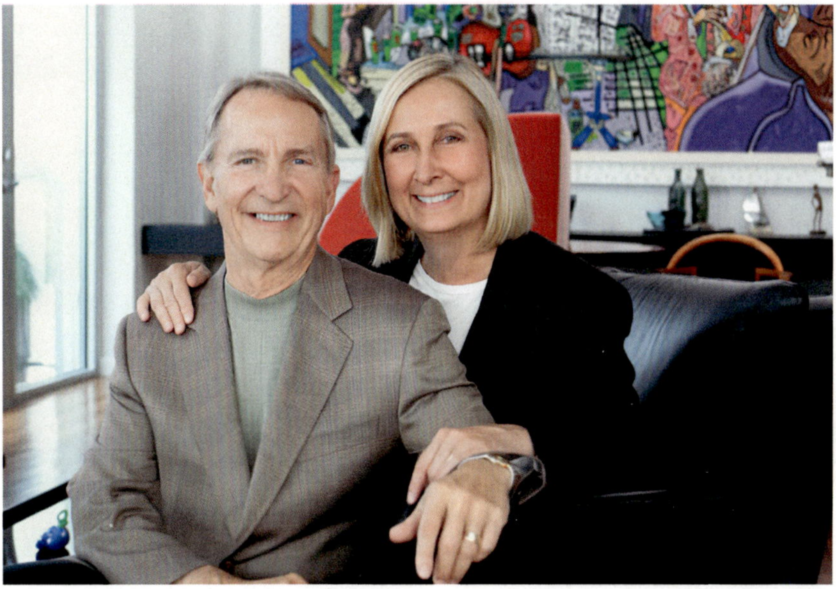

Jack Kearse/Emory University

Discovered bliss

My personal jury that has deliberated the existence of God for several years now has yet to issue a final verdict, but should they surprise me with an affirmative conclusion, I could only accept that if allowed to define the Supreme Being as the New Testament writer, Saint John, did; "God is love," he proclaims. I learned that from an avowed atheist.

I must have been deep in the throes of a preteen attempt to adjust to a new farm life near Nashville when Arlene Audray Stecenko presented herself to a Ukrainian immigrant father and a first-generation Polish mother on September 28, 1950, probably a cool day in Winnipeg, Manitoba, Canada. If there was something supernatural about the convoluted course each of our lives took toward their intersection three decades later, such a force moved in mysterious ways and took its own sweet time. If the outcome was inevitable, dictated by a prescient being with concerns for the happiness and welfare of earthlings, why let wanderlust and other intrusions delay things? Life, best lived, is patently too short for such distractions. But that seems to be the way things go. Makes me think we are pretty much left to our own devices without a lot of help from elsewhere. No cosmic GPS to expedite the trip. Too bad. Could have saved us a lot of time discovering the gifts of happiness and joy that love brings to mortal connections at their deepest and most consuming.

But we wandered. After graduating from medical school in Winnipeg, Arlene went to Australia for five years of additional training. I followed med school with stints in Baltimore, Phoenix, and San Francisco, eventually winding up back in Nashville for an almost thirty-year career that took me on numerous jaunts around the world on the pretense of advancing access to medical knowledge that was not readily available everywhere. Arlene arrived in Nashville because her then-husband chose to come there to study neonatology and she had agreed that it was his turn to choose their next assignment. She joined the unit I directed because I had a vacant position and she was interested in lung research, which was my unit's *raison d'être*.

So, near the end of a long, sometimes arduous, and inexplicable path, Arlene and I first met in my office at Vanderbilt to arrange for her two-year fellowship. We were both married to other people at the time, a significant deterrent to anything personal. She finished her fellowship, demonstrating excellent academic potential, and moved on with her husband to the faculty at the University of Florida where she continued her efforts to build a career. It was a few years before she ended her marriage and a few more years before I did the same. Eventually Arlene and I crossed paths again and discovered something new and precious about the potential of human relationships. We discovered love.

"If you don't believe in God," I asked her once, ruminating on her firm conviction that humanity is what it is and has neither need for nor evidence of a higher being hanging 'round to call the shots, "what is the point? What are we doing here?"

With barely a moment's pause, she replied, "To love and be loved."

I wrestled with that concept for a while—godless love challenged my youthful indoctrination, and I was not entirely free of that experience. But the ensuing years of peace, contentment, joy, and well-being that have bonded Arlene and me together with a sometimes-frightening intensity pull me in that direction. Maybe God is not love but love is God.

Early on in our relationship, I think on a moonlit night at her prairie home in Florida, we stood in the front yard thinking and talking. I was feeling insecure and was reacting to that by trying to convince Arlene that our relationship was not going to work, desperately hoping that my efforts would fail and that she would respond with a resounding declaration of her enduring love for me. She sort of did that.

"I can imagine growing old with you," she said, looking off into the distance at the rising moon and probably listening to the lowing of the cows out on the prairie.

We have aged together. Biology has a way of imposing chronology on us humans that is impossible to either ignore or escape. But "growing old is not for sissies" as Bette Davis is supposed to have said. Arlene has saved my life on more than one occasion when I am convinced that no force other than love could have done that. She has out-loved the mortal threats of cancer, heart disease, and other scary vagaries of innate human frailty.

So, what do we make of that, Saint John?

Knowing Cold

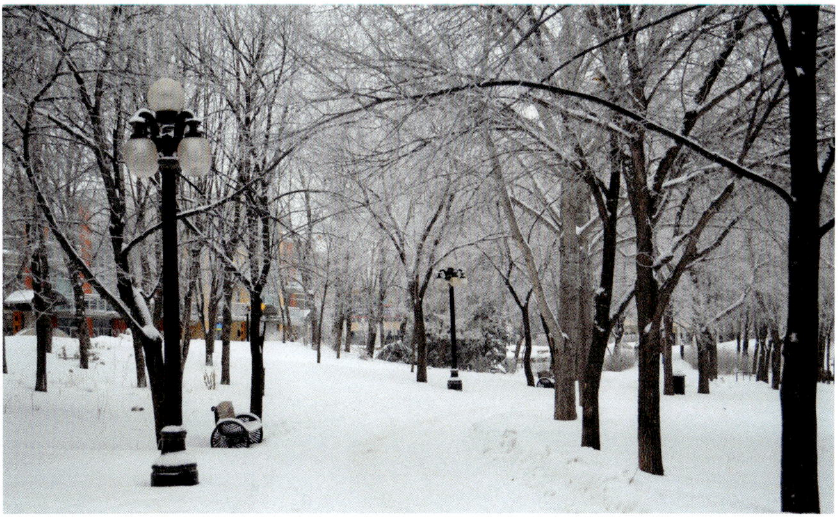

David Mark/Pixabay

Winnipeg in winter

You don't know cold until you spend a Christmas in Winnipeg.

I thought I knew cold. I had come to grips with both the concept and the reality in the winter of 1951 in Scottsboro, Tennessee, at the tender age of twelve, trying hard to adjust to the rigors of farm life without central heating, indoor plumbing, or running water.

Beginning on January 28 of that year with a light snow, the gods of inclement weather proceeded over the next several days to bless Nashville and its surroundings with a triple decker—an inch of ice, covered by a foot-thick blanket of snow, topped off by several more inches of ice. Temperatures plunged to twenty-plus below zero, and blizzardly winds stripped the landscape of most anything upright. Trees fell like toothpicks. Power lines scattered themselves across the countryside like so much spilled spaghetti, hissing and popping their electric threats and flash-frying any stray warm-blooded animal that wandered into them. The cold penetrated to my very bones and set up camp there until the weather broke after a week or two. I don't remember how long it took for me to thaw out, but it seemed like an eternity. I am still cold-natured. I often battle Arlene for control of the thermostat.

So, several decades later when I agreed to spend a Christmas in Arlene's hometown visiting her family, I had no qualms about facing a Canadian winter. I thought I knew cold. I was confident that the still vivid memory of my childhood encounter with extreme weather prepared me for such things. After all, how cold could it be?

The answer was very cold, as in a nadir of forty or more below on a good day, with temperatures wandering about deep in the world of negative degrees through day and night. The weather report on the radio gave statistics like how many seconds it was possible to stay outside without sustaining serious damage to exposed skin. And the locals appeared to assume that temperatures were destined to remain below zero. That's just what happened in Winnipeg wintertime.

"It's going to warm up today," someone said. "Radio says up to twenty."

I was elated until I realized that they meant a high of twenty below.

Cold and *white*. Winnipeg was disturbingly white that Christmas, all color frozen out of it and, for good measure, covered over by a lightning-white shroud of powdery snow. We're talking serious white. Moby Dick white. To venture into the outdoors was to be assaulted by bone-chilling cold that could be tolerated for only a few minutes and the painful glare of a world of unimaginable white that would have been excellent material for Ishmael's albino whale-inspired treatise on the subject.

We were staying with her mother in the house where Arlene had lived during much of her youth. A lot of togetherness. At one point during the visit, overcome with cabin fever, Arlene and I decided to take on the elements and stroll around a block or so, check out the old neighborhood. The elements won that battle. We made it a few yards down the street before we were forced to return to the warmth and color of Arlene's ancestral home. When compared to other possibilities, togetherness can have a positive side.

Warmth and *color*. After Arlene's father died her mother took up quilting. She discovered a flair for colors and patterns and became something of a virtuoso of the craft. Her quilts were works of art. Several of them were displayed about the house. There was at least one on every bed and several others scattered around to be used as coverlets in the living room and in the downstairs den. The colors and patterns of Mother Stecenko's handiwork added to the warmth of her house and were a welcome contrast to the bleached white out-of-doors.

The time arrived for the Christmas holiday celebratory family dinner, to be hosted by the people Arlene's brother, Richard, dubbed "the battling Bobyks." These were multiple generations of the progeny of Auntie Ida (Arlene's mother's sister) and Uncle Pete, her Ukrainian husband. There were quite a few of them, far outnumbering the paltry Stecenko contingent even if you included me and Lorna (Richard's wife). The dinner was to be held at one of the Bobyk's homes. I wasn't sure which one. There seemed to be several possibilities.

I dressed in all of the clothes I had managed to pack into my rollaboard. Even carefully layered and cinched up tight, they were insufficient. I thought that it was probably not possible to pile on enough clothes to make the weather tolerable, but I gave it my best effort. Feeling as overstuffed as the Pillsbury Doughboy, I heaved myself awkwardly into the rear seat of Ms. Stecenko's aging Oldsmobile for the short trip to the designated Bobyk domicile and a Christmas dinner with a gaggle of Canadians whom I had never met and, as it turned out, would never see again. Love is, on occasion, a demanding taskmaster.

The hosts had set up several folding tables in their thankfully warm basement to create a venue that could accommodate the sizable group. As the guests congregated, I was impressed with their apparent need for conversation and with their enthusiasm for the spoken word. For the most part I had no inkling of what was being talked about with such vigor—names I didn't recognize, incidents I knew nothing of recalled to gales of laughter. I just smiled self-consciously and swallowed another substantial draught of a citrusy white wine.

I was treated warmly enough but without a lot of empathy. I was, quite obviously, an intruder. And neither I nor the chattering Bobyks seemed highly motivated to change that. These people had a long and obviously cherished history to which I was not privy. I also got the feeling that Arlene may not have been their favorite relative. And taking up with an ethnically ambiguous divorced American ten years her senior from the U.S. South who knew nothing of East European culture, probably did little to enhance her standing with her extended family. At least that was my impression.

The meal was a Ukrainian-North American chimera. There was the familiar turkey and mashed potatoes. But also *golubtsi* (cabbage rolls) and probably *pirogue.* (I don't remember if that was so, but I ate a lot of those filled pastas during the visit. They seemed to be an essential part of most of these peoples' meals and I developed a serious taste for them.) The food appeared in waves of heaping dishes to the delight of the apparently ravenous Bobyks. The food was good, hardy fare that catered well to vigorous appetites, including my own. Perhaps there is something about intense cold and blinding white that stimulates the need for food. Maybe some kind of human survival advantage etched indelibly, eons ago, into our genomes.

The Oldsmobile yielded up its life to the bitter cold. As we prepared to leave, someone went to start the car so that it would warm up for our trip home. But, alas, the motor was as soundless as the snow-insulated late night and activating the starter had no noticeable effect. Mr. Olds' invention had been silenced by the force of nature. The situation was not in the least surprising to the Canadians; happened all the time. Just leave the keys with the host Bobyks, hitch a ride home with Richard and Lorna, and tomorrow someone would jump start the car and deliver it to Mother Stecenko's house. In the winter, Winnipegians become impressively creative and generous problem solvers. They have to be. Maybe the less creative ones are selected out, shipped off to warmer and less demanding places.

Why do human beings choose to live in such inhospitable places? Why did Natalie Asadchuk and her newly immigrated Ukrainian husband, Pete Stecenko, choose to settle down in Winnipeg, Manitoba, Canada and raise their two children there through many bitter winters to adulthood? Why did Richard Stecenko, Arlene's brother, a brilliant intellectual (his IQ probably hovers around 150) choose to live his life in his hometown until well into his seventies before leaving for a mellower climate on Vancouver Island? What is it about place that anchors many of us so firmly to a specific location on our planet?

Although the intensity of the bond to a specific place may suggest something pathologic, an Ahab-like obsession with a connection that tethers us to the vicinity of an especially meaningful spot, I don't think that's it. I also do not think it is a fear of adventure. Richard has traveled all over the world and sought out unusual experiences. (He once spent some weeks at a frozen camp in the Canadian North learning how to construct an igloo.) I think that some of us happen to have a snippet of DNA that defines us as *place people*. Most of the Havasupai, clinging desperately for generations to their beautiful but demanding home at the bottom of the Grand Canyon, must be driven by that special snippet. A lot of the mysteries of human behavior may be explained by how we happen to be wired.

Dying Fast

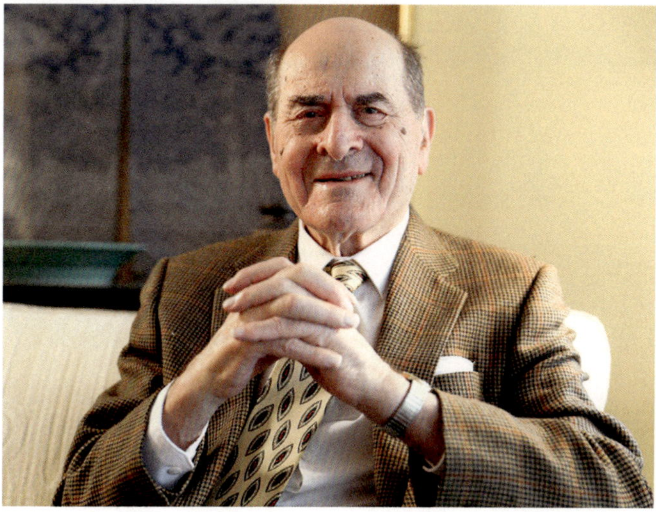

Henry Heimlich: Curer of the café coronary

My accidental friend, co-author (see *Predictive Health*, Basic Books, and *The Good Doctor*, Seven Stories), and very smart man, Mike Johns, reckons that what he calls the *square wave life*—stay pretty much healthy until near the end and then get the dying part over with as quickly as possible—is the ideal pattern for dealing with one's too brief time spent shuffling through this mortal coil. Although it was not intended, I came close to doing just that, i.e., getting the dying part over with quickly ... and prematurely. The personal consequences of almost dying, if it happens very fast, don't amount to much except on contemplation (dying slowly is another matter to be mentioned later on), but the actual event can attract yours and others' attention and certainly can intrude unpleasantly on an otherwise lovely dinner.

Although we no longer indulge the weakness very often, both Arlene and I have always liked red meat. Sit us down in a nice restaurant, serve us a well-chilled dry Plymouth gin martini (stirred) and then present us a bottle of a hearty cabernet and a thick slab of rare beef and we will smile at each other and at the pleasantness of life. We were doing that one fine evening at the now defunct Stockyard Restaurant (it was in what had been the Nashville stockyards) when suddenly and without warning, a bite-sized morsel of meat decided to lodge itself in the entrance to my windpipe instead of wending its way down my esophagus, the normal pathway for a masticated morsel of meat.

I could not breathe. I could not take in even the smallest amount of life-sustaining oxygen no matter how hard I strained. My eyes bulged. My skin went pale. I was aware that I might be dying, but I had no near-death experience as is sometimes described (my life did not parade across my consciousness; I made no rash promises to the Almighty in exchange for surviving this thing). All that mattered at that instant was that I could not breathe and every fiber of my being for a few moments was concentrated on that fact.

I have been repeatedly impressed with simplicity as a source of pleasure, creativity, achievement, and equanimity in the lives of human beings. (Heather once attributed to me a statement that I am not sure I made but with which I agree: *Life doesn't have to be complex to be extraordinary.*) So, it is surprising that it took the medical profession until 1974 to invent the cure for what had come to be known as the *café coronary* (which happens in cafes all right but has nothing to do with heart attacks; it's just that it happens so suddenly and kills so often, not to mention the appealing alliteration, that the term caught on). Surprising, because the rationale is so simple and the maneuver that cures it is so incredibly intuitive. Something is stuck in a tube. Raise the pressure beyond the obstruction suddenly and dislodge the thing. Dr. Heimlich figured that out and developed the maneuver that bears his name.

A youngish man in a dark blue business suit and a bright red tie with little figures on it arose calmly from his seat at the next table, positioned himself behind me, put his arms around my chest, interlaced his fingers and delivered a mighty heave, compressing my chest and raising the pressure in my windpipe (below the place where the offending morsel had lodged). Out popped the deceptively benign looking little gobbet, and as suddenly as I had almost died, I was entirely back to normal. I do not know who my savior was. He returned calmly to his dinner companions without speaking. I hope I at least bought him a drink.

Arlene was a nervous wreck for the rest of the evening. I calmly finished my steak and wine. I guess almost dying fast affects others more than the one doing the dying—at least at the time.

I had lunch once with a one-hundred-year-old woman who had numerous health difficulties (including surviving cancer). She said that she wanted to die suddenly, "but not yet." Maybe that's how it goes. You can accept the inevitability of the fact but would like a lot of liberty in choosing the timing. Personally, I want to live every day I am given, to delay starting the process of dying as long as possible. But once the inexorable process is underway, I think I'd like it to proceed pretty expeditiously. Give me long enough to say goodbye and every other unsaid thing that I can think of to the people I care most about. Please let me keep a reasonable amount of my wits and as much as possible of my dignity to the bitter end. And if it's not asking too much, let me keep my bodily parts functioning well enough that I can continue writing something useful until the words are gone, exhaled in my agonal gasp.

The Rule of Manuel

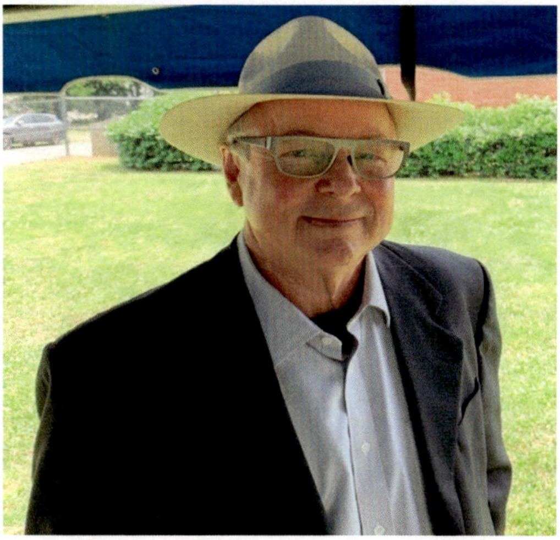

Courtesy of Manuel Zeitlin

Manuel Zeitlin: he of the eponymous rule

Manuel Zeitlin doesn't confront the world like most of us. He sees what can be, not what is. And he knows how to make it happen, how to summon new realities forth from old ones. Maybe that's what all architects do, but Manuel seems particularly good at it.

"Lights," we said to him. "We need more lights, but we're not sure where to put them, where they would fit into the decor."

"I would suggest," Manuel replied, *"that you put them where you want the light."*

He must have smiled although I don't recall whether he did. No matter. As he designed the renovation of our Printers Alley loft in Nashville, his rule often recurred in one form or another—*If it weren't there would you have put a fountain in the middle of your living room? And the mural of Fort Nashboro, pride of the previous owner, would you have had that painted on the wall by the bar?* The *Rule of Manuel* is deceptively simple, and witheringly obvious, in retrospect.

Probably in ignorant violation of the rule, we bought the loft apartment in Printers Alley, a down-on-its-heels Nashville night life area. An unusual address for professors in the medical school, but we were attracted to its authenticity. It was a real place, whether or not you liked the reality. A refreshing contrast to the insularity of the academic ivory tower. We had some lawyer neighbors who had presumably chosen to locate their business close to a primary source of customers. Denizens of the alley not infrequently found it necessary to seek legal counsel. For the most part, they weren't bad people, just occasionally found themselves crosswise with the law and needed some expert help.

When we decided that the loft needed some serious renovation, we invited Manuel and his lovely and equally talented wife, Janice, over for a drink hoping to interest them in the project. Drink sometimes helps in an effort like that.

"Rusted metal," Manuel declared.

We were sipping martinis and chatting about what I don't recall, but whatever it was, it had nothing to do with rusted metal. Manuel sat facing the elevator which opened directly into our living room, the shaft poorly disguised with a covering of some kind of drab brown paneling. It was not a very attractive centerpiece for the room. Manuel's creative juices must have roiled at the sight. His thought was to cover the entire thing with panels of rusted metal and he felt compelled to declare that on the spot unconcerned by the incongruence. (I don't think congruence was high on Manuel's personal priority list.) We eventually did the rusted metal and it worked well—elegance summoned forth from mediocrity for the price of a dry martini. There were numerous flashes of architectural brilliance on display in our eventually renovated flat. We finally had to abandon it as our jobs took us to Atlanta, but I was forever impressed with the influence of beauty on one's enjoyment of built space.

How does one discover exceptional talent, ferret out those few with *the gift*? Largely by accident, I think. We discovered Manuel and Janice first at Zeitgeist, the art gallery/salon that Janice ran at the time. She chose to handle mostly local artists of exceptional promise and, given her unusual ability to identify talent, probably played a major role in creating a market for Nashville art. Arlene and I patronized that market over the years. And we discovered Manuel.

Manuel's architectural business was also headquartered at Zeitgeist; we discovered his profession and met him on our first visit there. Arlene and I had been fretting over the light placement thing and thought he might be willing to help. Of course, he did that, but we also discovered that Manuel was a rising star in the local Nashville development community. He went on to play a major role in the renaissance of the city that continues to the present. Not only did he mastermind the renovation of our Printers Alley place, but we became enduring friends.

Friendship. How does it happen? What keeps it up? Why does it last?

Here's to the happy accidents of life and human nature that stage those special encounters.

And to dry martinis.

GeneRx, Inc., and the Maylie Bed

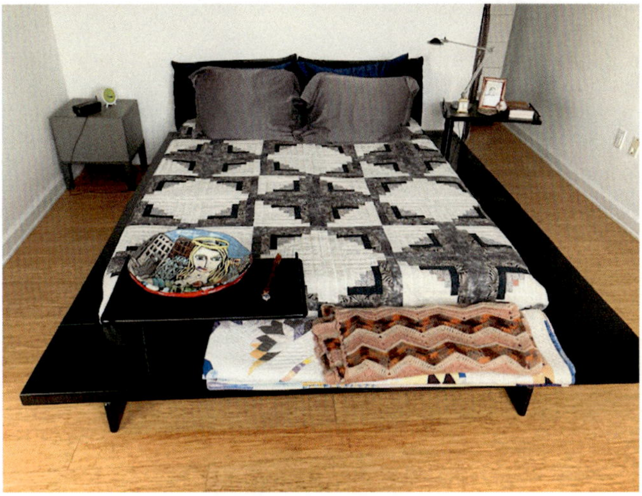

Author

The Maylie bed in situ

Mark Manner is near the front of the sizable collection of smart men I have had the privilege of knowing. And he and Anne are among the most interesting and charming couples on the planet (at least the parts of same that Arlene and I inhabit). We met them on a Sunday afternoon over our recently acquired Maylie bed.

We were attracted to the bed by the broad wooden surround, the multiple headboard pieces that could be inserted anywhere around the bed's perimeter, and the built-in bedside tables. The designer Peter Maylie created the special bed and it was very difficult to find in Nashville. We were finally able to order one through the Zeitgeist Gallery. Apparently, Mark and Anne (complete strangers to us at the time) happened into the gallery, struck up a conversation with Janice, and the topic of the Maylie bed cropped up. The Manners had been looking for one. Janice told them that we had bought the bed and that she was sure we would be happy to show it to them.

So, on a sunny Sunday afternoon, we had a call from Mark asking if he and Anne could come by our place to see if the bed they had fallen in love with from a catalog was up to their expectations. It was, but the generations-long saga that was triggered that afternoon has little to do with the reason for our meeting.

After showing them the bed, convincing them that it was just the ticket, we had a glass of wine and talked for a while. It turned out that Mark was a lawyer, a partner in a major local business law firm. It also happened that Arlene and I had just formed a small biotech company (GeneRx) based on our work on gene therapy for lung diseases at the university. We were totally naive about the mechanics of forming and operating a company. The company idea sprang from the need for funds to support our research and the availability of small business grants from the National Institutes of Health. We had experience with the NIH, but business-wise we were flying blind. Mark was just the expert we needed. He amazed me by offering to help us get off the ground. He more than kept that promise, shepherding us through the next few years pro bono. Alas, the enterprise eventually failed—poor timing, unforeseen events in the field, and probably our lack of business skills. Even Mark couldn't make up for that. But during those few heady years, Mark and Anne became dearest friends and are still.

That friendship led us into some adventures that we would not otherwise have been a part of. For example, we accidentally ran the Venice marathon. We just happened to be in the neighborhood, and it seemed like a good idea late at night after a dinner and perhaps a dram or two of wine to cloud our judgement. We had not signed up for the race, but somehow Mark discovered where it began and ended and arranged for a water taxi to pick us up early the next morning and transport us to the start line.

None of the four of us had trained for a marathon and coupled with the late evening, none of us was in optimal shape the morning of the race. But, to my surprise, we rolled out of bed, donned our running gear and headed for the hinterlands where the race began. Of course, none of us could run that far at any pace and so we missed the thrill of running over the pontoon bridge from Dorsoduro to Saint Mark's Square to collect a T-shirt memento. But we somehow arrived back at the flat we were renting only a little worse for wear. What are friends for if not to stress one's envelope of life experiences? There are a lot of other examples of Manner-devised adventures—*Mannerisms* maybe?

As I write this, I am still baffled by this friendship. I'm okay with the accident that started the whole thing—after all, my life has been largely directed by accidents. But what about that initial encounter planted such deep roots and nurtured them over the years? Is there something to the idea of chemistry among humans that intervenes to create intense and enduring connections? Is the whole process out of control, at least the control of those involved? I fear that I'm dangerously close to blaming the whole thing on fate or destiny or God or whatever you want to call some guiding force that runs the whole show. But I seriously doubt that is the case because it doesn't make sense to me. Mark and Anne may have been gifts to us from out of the blue, but I'm certain they would agree that it happened without any input from a force superior to human nature. Just doesn't make sense. It was probably the Zeitlins' fault.

The Rule of the Cashmere Peacoat

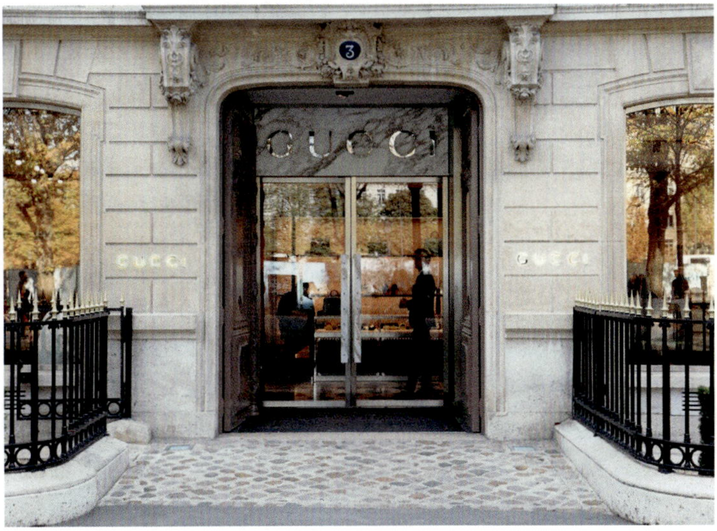

J Poulssen/Alamy Stock Photo

A Gucci boutique in Paris: Whence the rule

Should you decide to visit Paris, avoid at all costs the expansive glass and steel and concrete monstrosity the Parisians know as La Defense. Unless forced by employers with little interest in the influence of esthetics on their employees' performance to venture to this fortress at the western margins of their fair city, I am sure that it would long since have been deserted, written off as a colossal mistake by city fathers who had hoped to tap into a nonexistent streak of French pragmatism. Arlene and I arrived there by accident and we didn't stay long.

Arlene wept. She doesn't do that often, but the shattering of her vision of a romantic Parisian holiday by a hotel room in La Defense that resembled more a Holiday Inn in Omaha than the quaint luxury of a boutique establishment that we had envisioned was too much for her generally stalwart emotional firewall to withstand. And so, she wept.

But not for long. Declaring that she would "not stay in this place," Arlene looked through the sheaf of carefully researched materials she had accumulated for the trip and identified what turned out to be one of the most elegant hotels in the world, the Du Vigny, just a block or so off the Champs-Élysée. It was more than a mite pricier than planned for, but then how do you price out a dream? We confirmed that they had a room available, bid a not so fond adieu to La Defense, and proceeded to bask in the luxury of the Du Vigny for the duration of our stay in the City of Light. I don't remember how much it cost, but memories of the hotel that was our home base for a special holiday that still bring us pleasure are worth whatever it was.

Experiences are more durable than things. Grieving over disappointment is fine, but you don't have to let it spoil a dream.

We ate. We drank. I had a memorable lunch of bangers and mash at the Chameleon, a small, out-of-the-way eatery that we happened upon around lunch time. The tastes linger yet. No one does mashed potatoes like the French. We went for a long run one morning in a driving rainstorm, laughing at our old sweatshirts and threadbare tights that must have offended the sensibilities of the fashion-conscious natives. I had a Cuban cigar with my martini at the bar in the Georges V (no longer an acceptable indulgence). And we spent hours just walking the streets, window shopping and imbibing the distinctive ambience of the city. If traveling to new places is an education, it is for me an education of the senses, a visceral experience, rather than a cerebral one.

Sometime during one of our excursions into the city, we rounded a corner near the Champs-Élysée and were confronted with the display window of a Gucci boutique. In the window was a mannequin wearing a cashmere peacoat, the most beautiful coat I had ever seen. I recalled from my youth the rough wool peacoats from the army surplus store that kept me warm during many a winter. So my perception of the Gucci coat may have been tainted by a bit of nostalgia, but it really was beautiful. I wanted it. I had never seen a comparable garment. The price tag was not so pretty, however.

I don't remember the price, but it seemed exorbitant to me and given our less than careful attention to our monetary resources during this trip, despite Arlene's enthusiasm for the purchase, I couldn't summon a rationalization sufficient to do the deal. We stood for a while staring at the window in rapt admiration of the one-of-a-kind jacket that I would always regret having passed on the opportunity to own and continued our afternoon stroll through the city, sadder if not wiser.

So, the *rule of the cashmere peacoat* as articulated by my soul mate, keen observer of human behavior and its consequences, goes something like this. When you happen upon a thing that seizes your imagination and there is a single chance to get it, go for it, throw all caution to the wind and do the deed. If you don't, you'll waste a lot of time and energy regretting that you missed the chance. And few things dilute the joy of living like missed chances.

As a Christmas present in my eighty-first year, I received a cashmere peacoat. What took her so long?

Earth Dragons

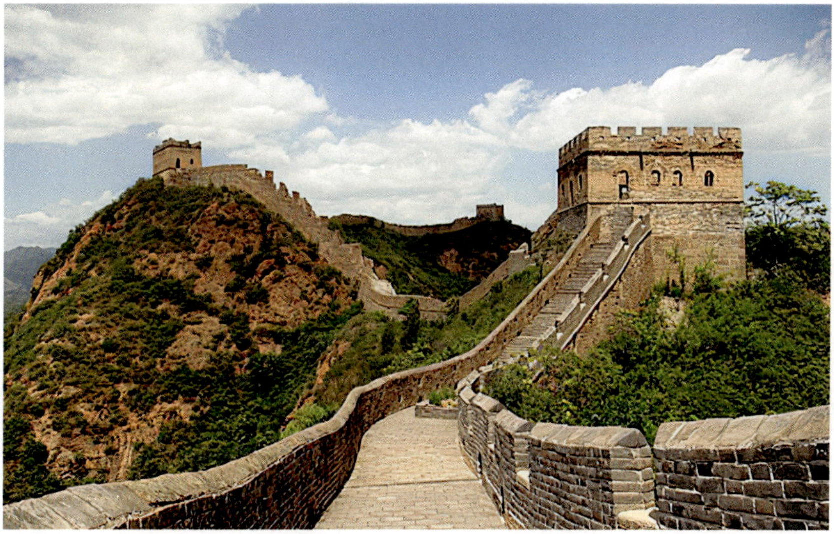

Jakub Hałun/CC BY-SA 3.0

The Great Wall of China

Poets have called it *Earth Dragon*, the iconic wall that snakes for more than ten thousand miles across the undulating Chinese borders from Liaodong in the east to Lop Lake in the west and from the Sino-Russian border in the north to the Tao River in the south. The wall has evolved over more than two millennia—possibly beginning as early as seven hundred BCE—into an architectural marvel that epitomizes the concept of a functional esthetic. It has resisted attempts at invasions by nomads from the Eurasian Steppe, permitted collection of fees for transporting goods along the Silk Road, allowed control of migration either in or out, served as a transportation corridor, and its watchtowers, barracks, and garrison stations have warned potential enemies for centuries of what any attempt to breach the empire's borders would be up against. A monument to power and beauty, the wall seduces both heart and mind. Of all the earth's marvels, you don't want to miss this one. If you do, your soul will be poorer for it.

A trip to China for Arlene and me, at the cost to us of making a few presentations to selected groups of medical professionals and students, came with a minder who kept a peeled eye on us pretty much all the time, but also served as a guide to, among other sites, the Great Wall. She rode with us on a hot, dusty day from Beijing to her chosen access spot at the wall and we climbed the steep bank of steps, shouldering our way through the crowd, to the crest. Even though there were solid stone steps, I felt the climb in my legs and lungs. It was that difficult.

But breathlessness and leg cramps aren't so important when you stand on top of the world. I was reminded of my first view of the Taj Mahal, confronting suddenly the devastating beauty of the place on passing through the marble gate. But this was different. The power and delicate beauty of this Earth Dragon floated off into eternity reflecting sensations that were difficult to fully comprehend and impossible to describe. Ghosts of pagan hordes from times past whose acquisitive ambitions were thwarted by the structure must still hang around to shake their spears in frustration at the gawking tourists. *If only*, they must echo ceaselessly into the vast ethereal space. As trite as the reaction is, it is impossible not to gawk.

Why Earth Dragon? Well, what better metaphor could there be than the beast that leads the New Year's parade and dominates the Chinese Zodiac. Endowed with awesome force and power, recipient of sometimes puzzling good fortune, driven by boundless energy, and focused with admirable tenacity on the task at hand, all tempered by a pervading sense of beauty and mystery, the Earth Dragon is easily seen as the personification of The Wall. At least so to a poet who envisions an anthropomorphic world.

Beijing duties done as best we could do them and the roles of American tourists played out to the apparent delight of our minder as well as ourselves, Arlene and I were off to Shanghai where a veritable thunder of Earth Dragons awaited us. Whoever the people were who shelled out a no doubt obscene number of yuans to finance this little jaunt wanted to extract as much value from our visit as possible and that meant assigning duties at each of their startlingly different major cities. We were delighted. What a bargain!

If you envisioned a traditional image of China, Shanghai would have startled you. There was little that felt like that China in the bustling center of commerce and social energy that struck the first-time visitor. Construction cranes swooped across the horizon piling tier upon tier onto emerging condominiums, office towers, and similar buildings, growing the forest of skyscrapers that defined the character of the cityscape. City streets pulsing with the thrust and parry of human life were lined with tony restaurants, elegant shops, trendy establishments that, except for their signs in Chinese, could have been in New York or Chicago or Atlanta. Our hotel felt familiar as upmarket hotels around the world tend to feel. We were entertained in a thirty-something floor condo near the city center. It was the residence of one of the physicians at the medical school where we were scheduled to lecture and was every bit as opulent and pretentious as the New York home of your generic Park Avenue plastic surgeon. Much about the city reeked of money, apparently excessive amounts of it.

Our invitation to China was initiated by a colleague at Vanderbilt where we were both members of the medical faculty at the time. The colleague was Chinese, on leave from his position on the faculty of the medical school in Shanghai, apparently one of the most outstanding Chinese medical institutions. Although we suspected that we had an unannounced minder while in the city, our colleague served as our visible host. Since neither Arlene nor I spoke Chinese, our host proposed to stand beside us on the stage as we presented and to translate the lectures for the audience.

That arrangement for the lectures was to my mind an unmitigated pedagogic disaster. Our slides were all in English and no doubt frustrated our host's efforts to translate and explain them to the audience. The translation was done pretty much sentence by sentence which hopelessly fractured any continuity to the narrative and protracted the time taken for the lecture to something approaching interminable. I did not see how anyone in the audience of advanced medical students could possibly have understood any substantial fraction of what was presented.

However, every one of the students, dressed in their Sunday best, sat alarmingly alert, raptly attentive, and giving every appearance of digesting each pithy morsel of the presented material. These were Earth Dragons—clever, bright, self-motivated, fortunate young people who were dedicated to their chosen task, overflowing with energy, and brimming with confidence. I had the feeling that someone in control must track the personal characteristics of their young and channel the Earth Dragons into medical careers. However these students were selected, they seemed to be a special group. Despite that, I am quite sure that Arlene and I did little to expand their medical knowledge. The language barrier, like the Great Wall, was probably impenetrable.

After one of the lectures, I asked a student how much he understood of what was presented.

"About ten percent" was his obviously strained response.

I had the feeling that the sentence contained a sizable fraction of the student's English vocabulary.

We left China, richer for the experience, but having failed, I fear, to earn our keep. We had taken much more than we had given.

Afloat in Sydney Harbor

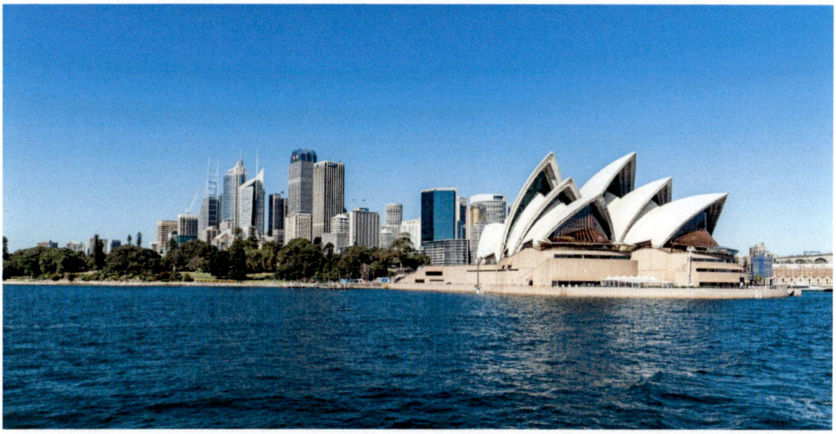

Llewellyn/Alamy Stock Photo

The view during lunch afloat Down Under

Arlene and I were drinking champagne and eating lamb chops like lollipops fresh off the charcoal grill mounted on the aft railing of an oceangoing sailing yacht anchored just across the harbor from the iconic Sydney Opera House. Brushstroke clouds smeared across the horizon beyond the cityscape seemed to capture the brilliance of the noonday sun and reflect it back onto the high-rise forest that spilled off to the side of the soaring wings of the opera house, backlighting the scene. It was something of a fortuitous homecoming for Arlene. She had left her hometown medical school in Winnipeg and spent several years of her medical training in Sydney and Melbourne. She had lived just across the harbor bridge from the city for a time and had many memories of the place.

We were guests, for the harbor cruise, of an affluent Australian doctor who was apparently enamored of the entertaining life as well as the sailing life. There were several other guests, all connected somehow to an international medical meeting to which I had been invited as a speaker. The sailing outing was one of several social occasions staged by the Australian meeting organizers. I got the impression that the meeting may have been mainly an excuse rather than a reason. Aussies are gregarious sorts and would scarce miss a chance for a party.

A warm, sunny afternoon spent on a leisurely sail about a scenic harbor that clung tightly to the underside of our planet was surely a pleasant enough use of one's time. Visitors from the upper latitudes settled easily into the comfort of the day—warm sun, good food, generous drink, the elemental sense of big water bearing up a sturdy boat—free of any need for explanations. We were there and, for the moment, that was good enough. There would be space for my professional performance later. If I needed to, I could contrive a reason for our being there that might be as true as the occasion required.

On a somber, gray morning, we jogged in a driving rainstorm along the crest of Mrs. Macquarie's Point out to its tip. We stood there for a time bathing in the warm rain and gaping at the panorama spanning the harbor from the bridge to the opera house. Centuries earlier, the wife of Major General Lachlan Macquarie, governor of New South Wales, would sit on the rocky prominence and watch for ships from Great Britain sailing into the harbor. Her husband had the stone sculpted into Mrs. Macquarie's chair that squats serenely on its haunches at the end of the point, still watching for ships from the motherland.

We spent a morning strolling through The Rocks and had lunch at a trendy restaurant that overlooked the harbor. Long gone are the traditional thatched roof houses of waffle and daub favored by aboriginals and others forced to the margins of the growing city; it was their sandstone replacements that gave the place its name. The Rocks was a rapidly gentrifying area, prime real estate on the water and close to the city center. Its checkered social history lent it local color that increased its allure to modern developers. Even down there in the earth's underbelly, in a country founded by criminals, the inexorable march of civilization proceeds apace. People are people and insist on being so regardless of where the fates destine them to make their place.

Dressed to the nines, Arlene and I sat in white-draped folding chairs set up on the grounds of a racetrack, enjoying our wine and the small band playing on a makeshift stage. Apparently Australians do this a lot, commandeer an idle racetrack as a venue for a celebration of some kind. I guess racetracks, like churches, have a lot of down time that can be put to good use. Well along in the evening's entertainment, the band struck up the distantly familiar strains of "Oh Julie," the vanilla rock hit from the fifties that was recorded by a group of which I was a member at the time. I'm not sure how they found out about that arcane bit of my history and less sure how they got the sheet music and staged this unexpected interlude, but they did. I was propelled by the applause of the crowd to respond to my introduction by the emcee by taking the stage and making a really sorry attempt to sing a verse or two of the song that I had long since forgotten. It was a truly terrible performance. As I walked back to my seat, I heard a woman say, "It's a good thing he chose to go into medicine." I heartily agreed with her sentiment as did, I suspect, the rest of the crowd who felt obliged to endure the spectacle. I appreciated the attempt at humor, but there are few things that disappoint me more than a poor performance.

I suppose that, stuck there on the earth's downside, Australians have learned to amuse themselves at the expense of outlanders from up top. A sense of isolation pervades the place that may strain any universal human ties that bind our species together. After all, they'll probably never see us distant outlanders again. May as well have a little fun.

Sidling Up to the Crab

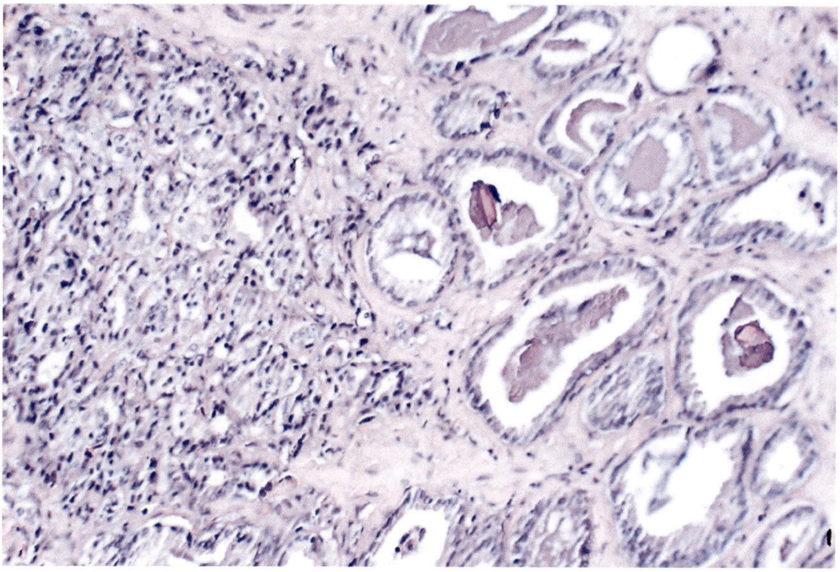

Otis Brawley/National Cancer Institute

Photomicrograph of the wicked wee beasties

Take cancer, for example ... mostly an accident as best I can tell. Granted, if you are morbidly inclined or tend sufficiently toward self-destruction, you can invite in the dreaded crab, roll out the red carpet—smoke a lot of cigarettes, lick the tip of the radium-laden brush you use to make the dial of a wristwatch glow in the dark, or drink water that is laced with the carcinogenic effluvium of industrial chemical plants. However (and I can personally vouch for the veracity of this statement) even if you don't do most of those things, you might still get cancer. I did. I discovered it quite by accident. It could have killed me in what, in retrospect, I consider the prime of my life, but for a purely serendipitous stroke of fortune.

Some deep background. If there is a hierarchy among male reproductive glands, the testicles are the alpha beast. That's where the fundamental business happens, where the stuff of future generations is made. The prostate gland is in the neighborhood, a friendly neighbor for the most part, patiently supplying the juice that the fecund squigglies need for swimming out from their gland of origin to their intended destination where the rest of the process gets underway. The prostate gland just sits there and makes more juice in case it is needed, a pretty much passive enabler of the alpha beast's intended actors. The great majority of these glands are perfectly happy with this less glamorous secondary role in procreation, completely comfortable with granting center stage to the neighboring testicles and their wriggling spawn, satisfied to just go about doing their job and not making any trouble. A reliably blue-collar sort of gland.

However, for every nine prostate glands that spend their entire lives like that, gladly playing the role of supporting actor, one will succumb to a lust for stardom. After sitting for perhaps decades resting quietly astraddle the urethra and attracting little attention, these suddenly overly ambitious glands manage to wrestle themselves free of the surly bonds of normal biology, bursting forth as full-blown cancers onto center stage, leaving in the wings the glitzier testicles to nurse their wounded egos. Cancers attract a lot of attention. The newly malignant prostate becomes for a time the most important gland in the entire body. Knives are whetted, an array of toxic chemicals is produced, big noisy machines are cranked up that generate ammo dumps—X-rays, protons—all focused laser-like on destroying the malignant gland, the consequences for the rest of the body be damned. Curing cancer is a messy business.

Here (at least in my case) we encounter a consequence of the life insurance industry's aversion to risk. That is not how things should have happened, but it's how they did.

I was a fifty-ish year old, well-educated and successful academic doctor. My father died of prostate cancer when I was a teenager and it was not pretty. I did not have fond memories of that process. So, I was familiar with the disease in both theory and practice. But I had given precious little thought to whether my very own prostate gland would betray me. I mean, I felt great. I wasn't doing much of anything risky (at least not cancer-risky). Contrary to what you might expect, given my family history, the inner shenanigans of that wrinkly little walnut sized morsel of a gland rarely crossed my mind. That is until I decided it was time to insure my life (an odd way to express it; life insurance actually insures one's death, not one's life, but that's another subject).

The people who sell you life insurance would prefer that you were immortal, in which case, of course, you wouldn't need life insurance at all. So before signing you up, they do everything reasonable to prove to themselves that you are as close to immortal as possible for a living human and so unlikely to avail yourself of the benefits of their product for the foreseeable future. For a middle-aged man, that includes drawing blood and measuring your Prostate-Specific Antigen (PSA), a protein that is thought to indicate the presence of cancer. Thus (I'm sure you have guessed already) they measured my PSA and it was high. Not astronomically high, but definitely high.

The terrible thing about numbers, especially numbers that are presumed to be relevant to your health, is that once you have them, you are stuck. Once done, it is not possible to unmeasure one's PSA (or blood sugar, hemoglobin A1c, C-reactive protein ... even weight for that matter). Once measured and found to be elevated, the burden of proof becomes yours. Guilty until proven innocent. If I were to get life insurance, it was up to me to prove that I did not have prostate cancer. I needed a letter from a qualified professional to the effect that I was cancer free.

That's where the fun started. To obtain such proof, one must enlist the aid of a urologist. Indignity is too mild a word to characterize what urologists do to their victims. Upon entering a urologist's exam room, one is obligated to remove one's clothes, of course, but also to divest oneself of any remaining shred of dignity that one had hidden away someplace, desperately hoping to hang on to it as a modicum of support for the impending urological ordeal. Forget it. The gloves are off (well, metaphorically, anyway; actually the surgeon's gloves are on and grasping a truly evil appearing instrument of impending torture). I'll spare you the details; I don't care to remember them. The biopsy was taken and proved to be negative. The doctor wrote the letter and I got the insurance.

But there is more to this story.

Urologists, bless their sadistic hearts, have great difficulty ignoring an elevated PSA, even after a negative biopsy. If it stays high, they are compelled to have another go at sampling the gland. More indignity. More yielding to their need for inflicting pain and humiliation. More waiting anxiously for the pathology reports. And, at least in my case, more negative results.

So, this whole scenario degenerated into a duel between my steadily rising PSA and my urologist's commitment to uncovering the chemical's malignant source. I, that is me as a person, was pretty much marginalized. The situation was out of my hands. This was now an existential battle of doctor vs. aberrant biology. A battle at the front lines of the war on cancer; in the trenches, so to speak. My presumed cancer would occupy center stage while the rest of me (you know, heart, soul, ethos, emotions, passions, desires, etc.) was pretty much incidental to what was going on. Take off your clothes, hang any remaining fragment of your dignity on the coat hook behind the door and bend over. We'll find this damn thing whatever it takes.

Well, he found it, but it wasn't easy. I was eventually anesthetized so the urologist could really get into the biopsying business, spared from my whining. The tissue indeed showed cancer which the urologist informed me of by phone a day before Arlene and I were leaving for a medical meeting in New Orleans. The next day was Mother's Day, which seems significant in my memory although I have no idea why. I don't see what celebrations of motherhood have to do with aberrant prostate glands. But then there are a lot of experiential connections that don't seem obvious until some genius sees them for what they are.

At the time one's best bet for curing a cancer like this was an operation called a radical prostatectomy. Given the appropriate anatomy, the operation cures the cancer based on the simple premise that if you remove all of the cancerous tissue, the thing will not recur. That is a simple enough premise, but it does not account for the undesirable consequences of the surgery—impotence and incontinence are real possibilities. So the decision to go for the surgical cure has implications that might involve the happiness and equanimity of others. Like I said earlier, curing cancer is often a messy business.

Arlene and I made the mutual decision that since my life was threatened, it was best to get rid of the offending tumor and deal with whatever happened to be the consequences. The surgical deed was done and I emerged cancer-free. We are still dealing with the complications several decades later, but I am alive and we are still in love. (I kept a journal during the ordeal that was published as *Hard Bargain* by Harpeth House Publishers.)

Change

The Implosion of a Sinecure

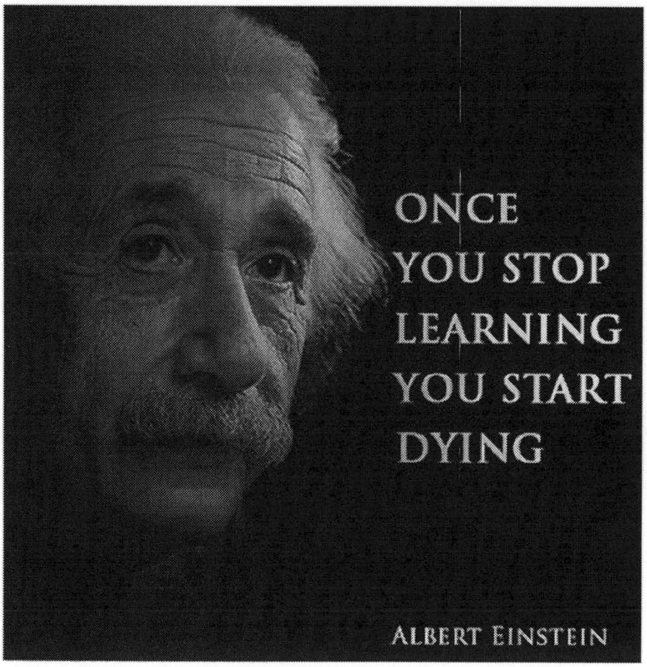

Internet Meme

After almost thirty years of serious commitment to and considerable professional accomplishments at what I had long considered my academic home, that institution made me the worst job offer that I could have imagined ... a sinecure.

The younger colleague to whom I had bequeathed my previous leadership role said (as I remember it) something like, "You can keep your office, your salary, and you don't have to do anything. How can you possibly beat that? Aren't we all aiming for a big salary and no responsibility? Well, you're there, Ken. Relax and enjoy it."

If there had been any remaining doubt in my mind about accepting the Vice Chair of Medicine job at Emory that I had been offered, that conversation would have erased it. True, I had been a tenured professor for many years and so, at least in theory, I couldn't be fired. But I was being offered a worse fate—a useless role explicitly created to expose the institution's conclusion that I no longer brought it academic value. Like the failed athletic coach, I was to be bought off and secreted somewhere in a little frequented part of the university to pass my remaining days recalling old glories and to wither away trapped in a developing shroud of cobwebs of obsolescence. "NO WAY!!" I was tempted to shout to the heavens.

I had long thought that the concept of tenure, while a well-intentioned intellectual construct, was a patent fiction. The idea of protecting our academic brain trust from administrative shenanigans that sometimes value truth and beauty less than they ought was meant, I guess, to enshrine institutions of higher learning as fortified bastions of social and intellectual integrity, gatekeepers of the academic soul. Hard to argue with that at least as a surface motive. The problem is that it doesn't work. It doesn't work because a lot of us are more attracted to the *tragedy of the commons* (consuming excessive amounts of common resources to the eventual detriment of us all) than to selfless nobility in our dealings with each other.

So, when I age, present me with a sinecure and I will either take it, relinquish any vestige of intellectual curiosity, park myself out of the way and get about the business of dying, or I will refuse to accept the notion that I am worthless and look for something productive to do. Neither does much to protect the integrity of the academy. For more determined managers, there are even better ways—reduce my salary, take away my office, make me generally *persona non grata* and I will leave one way or another. Tenure doesn't protect me from being fired, although it may influence the process. Whatever the motives of the new generation of leaders at my hallowed institution for wanting to rid themselves of an aging tenured faculty member who was no longer valued, I am sure that they didn't have to ponder the tactics for very long. People in managerial positions at leading organizations learn those things somewhere very early in their ascent to leadership.

In fact, the lives of our academic institutions and even of its aging faculties may have been saved by the emasculation of tenure. Maybe ecclesiastical positions "without the care of souls" (*sine cura*) that originated the idea had some constructive function, but divorcing responsibility from reward runs a serious risk. The nineteenth century Scottish police reformer Patrick Colquhoun thought so—"Many of the best institutions moulder into sinecures," he wrote. I think that also happens to individual people who rest too firmly on their accumulated laurels and don't ask questions anymore. I don't think mouldering is very constructive for either people or institutions, but sometimes neither has the perception and energy to avoid that fate. Maybe better to do away with the temptation.

So probably to the bafflement of my productive and curious younger colleagues and no doubt others whose life goals were skewed by a misperception of the opportunities that age presents, I refused a sinecure. I am not mouldering and steadfastly refuse to do so. I am as curious as I ever was although the targets of my curiosity are more inclusive than they once were. And I use different tools to spelunk in the caves where the mysteries of life that intrigue me lie unexplored.

Life didn't come with tenure. We must have invented the concept as a futile attempt to avoid dealing with the finality of it all. The end is always near and getting closer. That was true from the start.

Carpe diem.

The Real Doc Hollywood

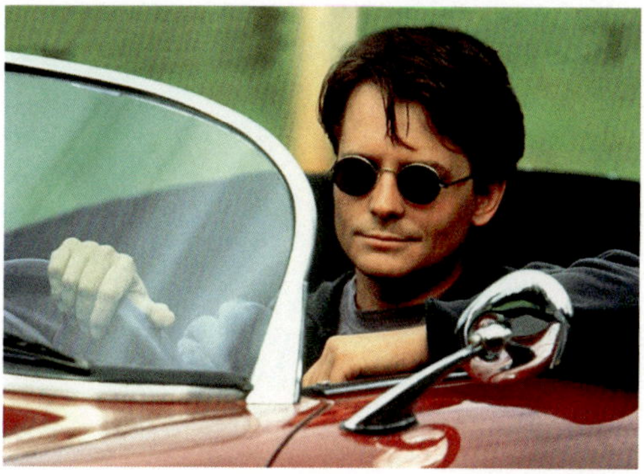

Allstar Picture Library Ltd/Alamy Stock Photo

Doc Hollywood (the movie version)

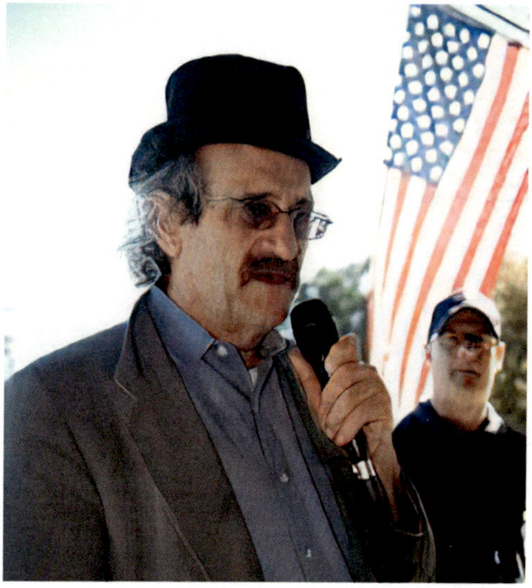

Kevin Trotman Photography (CC BY-NC-ND 2.0)

The Real Doc Hollywood

I know as an absolute certainty that Michael J. Fox is not the real Doc Hollywood; he just played the role in a movie. And M.J.F. bears precious little personal resemblance to Neil Shulman, MD, the real-life doctor, standup comic, and author who wrote the book and helped produce the movie. I met Neil over the cheese board at an Emory University Department of Medicine Christmas party. The man gravitates to food.

He wore tattered tails, a threadbare red vest, and a lopsided top hat perched precariously atop his Einsteinian nest of unruly gray hair. He looked hopelessly out of place among the staid group of well-coiffed, sedately clad doctors and other health professionals, but it was obvious that he was unconcerned about that. Neil is comfortable in whatever space he finds himself, especially if there is food to be had. He is a garrulous sort and my interest in writing led us into a conversation about how he happened to morph a few years earlier into his current persona from a New York-to-Atlanta transplanted physician who spent his time caring for a mostly minority population of people with high blood pressure. I was really interested in how one goes about accessing the ponderous machinery of the publishing world given my aspirations along those lines. Neil wasn't a lot of help.

However, he did stimulate me to actually write something, got me started again. He had written a screenplay, a somewhat bizarre story about a weird psychiatrist, a medical student, a goldfish named Einstein, and some other stuff, and asked me to write it into a novel. I did that (we self-published the novel under the title *Spotless*). We co-authored another novel after that (*The Asolo Accords*, also self-published). Although those efforts were not among my best, they got me started doing something I enjoy that has kept me busy during my retirement from medicine. If you have any doubts about the role of accidents or serendipity or whatever in the direction of one's life, I raise my completely unexpected encounter with the real Doc Hollywood at the Christmas party cheese board as pretty solid evidence for it. Even now, Neil always shows up when I have a book signing, especially if there is food.

I would guess that Neil's Jewish grandmother in New York was less than thrilled with how he turned out. After all, he went to the trouble to become a doctor, a profession considered by many to be about as good as one is likely to do. Why head off in another direction?

My theory is that both performers and writers are born, not made, and Neil was born that way.

"How do you know if you're a writer?" I asked a knowledgeable person once.

"If you write," he answered.

The same could be said of performing, and even if you don't do either very well, the urge can be irrepressible. Neil has written numerous books, some alone and more often with a co-author. True, they mostly have a medical slant, but after all, that is what he knows—*write what you know* the advisors say.

Neil keeps a loose connection with medicine. When given the chance, he stands up and tells jokes. He plays the clown in public with equanimity. And he writes. Neil is fine with that. Sorry, Grandma.

Martinis with Ghosts at the Golden Dove

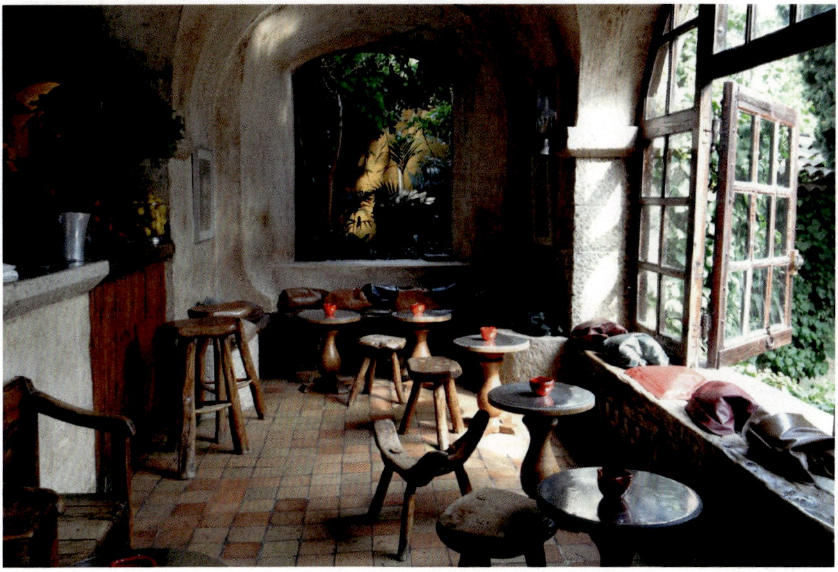

Photo (c) Janet Minker

The bar at the Colombe d'Or

What hallows a place?

We sat at the small bar in the Colombe d'Or sipping martinis. I was studying a signed photograph of Pablo Picasso hanging inconspicuously beside where I sat and thinking about the ghosts of the artists, intellectuals, and the odd glitterati who had passed through there and left their tracks. Yvonne Roux, aging consort of the ghosts, graced the bar with her presence. Arlene and I chatted with her a bit about the history of the small hotel and of Saint Paul d'Vence, the Cote d'Azur town whose walls loomed gently over the Golden Dove and its surroundings, forever haunted by the dazzling ghosts of genius.

"Was Picasso surprised by his fame?" I asked.

"Oh, heavens no," Madame Roux replied. "He felt it was overdue and insufficient to his talent. They were mostly like that—Miro, Braque, Chagall. And later, Calder, Cesar, and the others."

Their names were all signed in the guest book and their art cluttered the place, many pieces used as payment for a stay at the hotel or a meal. Tracks of the ghosts of genius etched in the amber realities of biology—rest, food. Dazzling.

I looked back over my shoulder at Picasso. I wondered: Are extraordinarily gifted people bound to an outsized perception of themselves, the gift and the person a fused organic whole like Siamese twins, mitosis halted at a critical point, before the separation was complete? Maybe so. Or maybe those guys (mostly guys) were just insufferably arrogant folks who happened, like idiot savants, to have fallen into the gift. Does that matter to the rest of us?

James Baldwin spent his final years in Saint Paul d'Vence and left some tracks there. Mr. Baldwin left a lot of tracks around the world that have etched deeper with the passing of time. Our connection with him was another accident, product of the inexplicable vagaries of life that involved James's younger brother, David. David was not well but still spent time at James's villa, a short distance down the hill from the Golden Dove. I'm sure both James and David had downed a libation or two at the bar there. The place was hallowed many times over. Destiny or caprice? Hard to tell. Does it matter to the rest of us?

David's significant other at the time lived in Vence and after meeting us at the bar, took us in tow for an afternoon and evening. We meandered with her down the serpentine lane that led to James Baldwin's villa and spent some time there. We lingered in the room where we were told that Baldwin finally died, a torrent of blood spewing forth from his gastric cancer. There was a box of vintage jazz LPs sitting in a corner. There were some collages on the wall, products of David's interest lately in that art form. Outside, the site of Baldwin's famous welcome table was barely identifiable, the space largely overgrown with weeds and such. Magic may be durable, but the world continues to turn and time tries hard to obscure the stuff that's hard to understand. Weeds where once the brilliant expounded over food and wine and the camaraderie of like-minded folk. The echoes persist but grow fainter. The world continues to turn and some things are still hard to understand. Human beings are not very reliable in the setting of history.

We were treated to dinner at a small café in Vence. Some jazz played softly in the background. I don't remember what we ate. We talked of the Baldwin legacy and reflected on the place, his place, shared with the host of exceptional people who had gravitated there over the years. Later we shared another drink with those ghosts.

A Flat in Venice

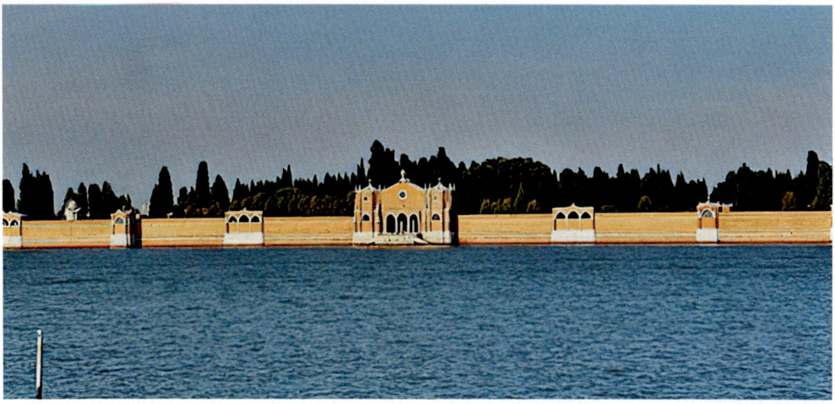

San Michele, the cemetery island, Venice

If you are not Italian and you take a foolish notion to buy a flat in Venice, you would do well to get to know Giorgio Crivelli—sculptor, electrical engineer extraordinaire, and secretly aspiring harpsichordist. He lives with his Venetian wife, Chiarina, in Milano, Venezia, aboard his yacht (*Agora*), and various other places as the mood strikes him. He pays his taxes in Switzerland because they are cheaper than in Italy, wishes his remains to be interred on San Michele, eternal island resting place for the Venetian elite, and liberally indulges his apparent penchant for helping other people realize their dreams. Giorgio Crivelli is an extraordinary man.

Arlene and I first visited Venice together on our way home from a medical meeting in Stresa, a charming waterfront village in the lake country north of Milan. She fell hopelessly in love with the city. Not everyone does, you know. Englishmen often complain of an unpleasant odor emanating from the canals. And there are the eternal parades of tourists from everywhere, frequent targets of complaints from both the few remaining locals and from other tourists. Also there is the summer heat, mosquitoes, and lack of air conditioning. Arlene didn't feel any of that. She absorbed the spirit of the place, the penetrating mystery and mesmerizing art and architecture that are the essence of the Venice soul. It was pure unadulterated love at first site.

After that visit, we resolved to return to Venice every year, renting an apartment and trying to live more like a local than a tourist, baptizing ourselves in the pure Venetian *acqua vita*. We did that, and after a few years, began to wonder if we could afford to buy a small flat there and whether the logistics would prove too daunting even if we could. Some Internet advertised prices for small apartments, studios mostly, looked encouraging pricewise. But how could Americans ensconced in their Atlanta condo and wedded to jobs at the University Medical Center go about navigating the vagaries that must be inherent in doing business in Italy long distance?

I resorted to contacting our one acquaintance who knew more about everything in the world (and beyond; he was an accomplished amateur astronomer) than anyone else I knew. I called Mark Manner. A total flyer. I had no reason other than my general observation of the breadth of his worldly knowledge that Mark would have any way to provide advice about this particular problem.

As a result of that call, we found ourselves guests of Giorgio and Chiarina Crivelli for a private lunch at the Venice Yacht Club, sitting on the sunny veranda and looking out over the Saint Mark's waterfront. It turned out that Mark's Nashville firm had done business with a London firm that had connections in Rome where Giorgio was a consultant for legal matters in his area of expertise. Mark was given contact information for Giorgio. We exchanged emails and were eventually invited to lunch the next time we were in the city. Giorgio had done some homework and had information about apartments that we could possibly afford. One was especially interesting.

Giorgio's friend, Morisin, an elite metal working artisan, had a shop in Cannaregio but lived with his wife outside the city. He had bought and renovated a ground level studio near his shop that looked out on the *fondamente nove*, across the lagoon to a face-on view of

San Michele, the cemetery island, as well as a view of the skyline of Murano in the distance. Morisin had decided to sell the studio, yielding to his wife's desire for a place in the Dolomites.

Our initial visit to the place was that very afternoon. After lunch, Giorgio joined us in the apartment we were renting and after consuming upwards of half a bottle of single malt Scotch, we discovered that Giorgio had brought the keys to Morisin's studio and he invited us to stroll down to the *fondamente* to see it. After a brief courtship with the possibility, we convinced ourselves that this was just the Venice place we were looking for.

And Giorgio, with considerable personal effort, arranged and executed the sale. He flew back from a business meeting in Rome solely to attend the closing. We joked after the lengthy meeting where the solicitor insisted on reading an endless Italian document of which we understood absolutely nothing that we had bought either ourselves or Giorgio a Cannaregio apartment. For several years now, the flat has been a frequent and very special retreat for us in the most beautiful city in the world and Giorgio and Chiarina have become fast friends.

Yet another example of an enigmatic path to friendship. How could anyone have predicted the convoluted path that led to this whole thing? In this case, my guess is that it was primarily the Crivellis' fault. They probably had thousands of friends because of who they are and we were lucky enough to drop into their orbit. They cared about people. And they were dream makers. We just happened to discover them and they did what they do—birthed one more dream and in the process added new friends to their ever-lengthening list.

Lunch With Palladio

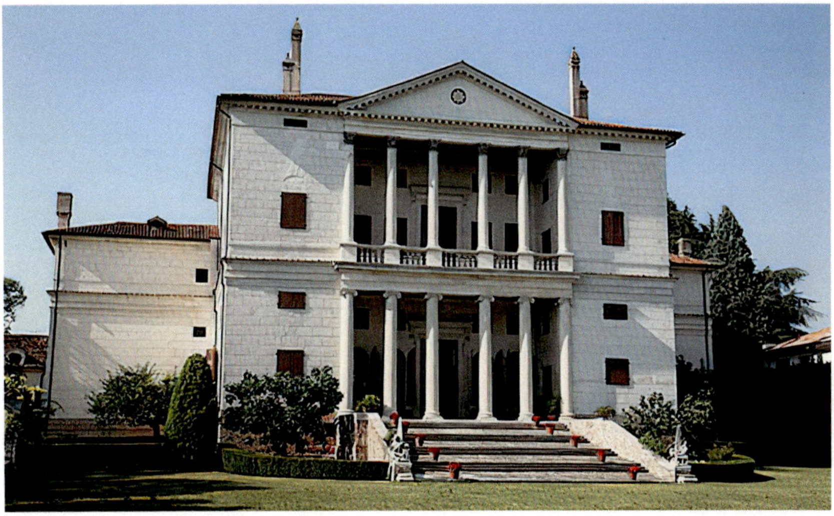

Villa Cornaro, Piombino Dese, Veneto, Italy

The central salone that anchors the grand symmetry of the Villa Cornaro, a mid-sixteenth century master work of the Italian Renaissance architect Andrea Palladio, echoed with the banter of a noted physics professor from nearby Padua, an American reporter with connections in Venice and his wife, and the rest of us—me, Arlene, and our gracious hosts, Atlantans Carl and Sally Gable. Arlene and I had made the short train ride from Venice where we were staying to Piombino Dese, the Veneto village where Giorgio Cornaro had commissioned Palladio to design and construct his summer retreat. Realizing a long incubating dream, Carl and Sally had bought the place and continued its restoration to something as close as currently possible to the villa where Signore Cornaro escaped from the worst of the searing Veneto summers.

How did we manage to get invited to such an elegant and interesting lunch by such elegant and interesting hosts? We had no personal connections in Venice; we just loved the place. Neither

Arlene nor I had ever met any of the other guests who were in Piombino Dese that sunny afternoon. In Atlanta, our modest circle of friends rarely impinged on the Gables' active social life. The email invitation appeared out of the blue and, even in retrospect, I am surprised that it came. It was almost certainly the Ingrams' fault.

We were invited to dinner at the Druid Hills home of Roland and Marguerite Ingram where we first met their friends Carl and Sally Gable, because the Ingrams had somehow discovered that we had fallen in love with Venice. Roland was a former professional colleague who had been retired for a while. He and Marguerite were an attractive couple who were fond of small dinner parties that included people who didn't know each other but who were judged by the hosts to be potential friends. They were probably delighted when their scheme worked. They had an enviable cadre of fascinating friends and must have enjoyed a hobby that was essentially rearranging relationships among interesting people. On that particular evening, the Ingrams' undivulged targets were me and Arlene and the Gables. Although it took a while, their effort was a resounding success.

Over several ensuing years, we were invited to the Gables' elegant Atlanta home for dinner, sometimes a small affair entirely arranged (and cooked for) by Sally and sometimes a large catered party of mostly people who, like the Gables, lived a tier or two higher on the socioeconomic scale than we did. Blessed with the imprimatur of the Gables, we always felt welcome on those occasions, regardless of whom was there.

Sally and Carl spent mostly summers in their Piombino Dese villa since the place was not heated. When our visits to Venice coincided with the Gables' presence, we often had lunch with them, sometimes at our modest studio apartment on the *fondamenta nove* and sometimes at a nearby restaurant. Carl was something of a Venetian scholar and his comments on the nature and history of the architecture as we strolled through the city added a new level of intellectual appreciation of the place that complemented what was for us a mainly visceral experience.

There was no real reason for us to know the Gables. Carl was retired from a position as chief executive of a sizable company and Sally was a gifted musician. We lived in different worlds for the most part. Those worlds were separate enough that had it not been for a shared love of things Venetian and the social creativity of the Ingrams, we would never have encountered each other—no lunches with Palladio for us.

Friendships, even accidental ones, can bring with them lessons about the inherent goodness of one's fellow humans that unlearned would make for a poorer life. Our lives are richer for having known the Gables. Palladio's handiwork contributed to that, but it was the connection with genuinely good people that mattered most.

Sutton Place

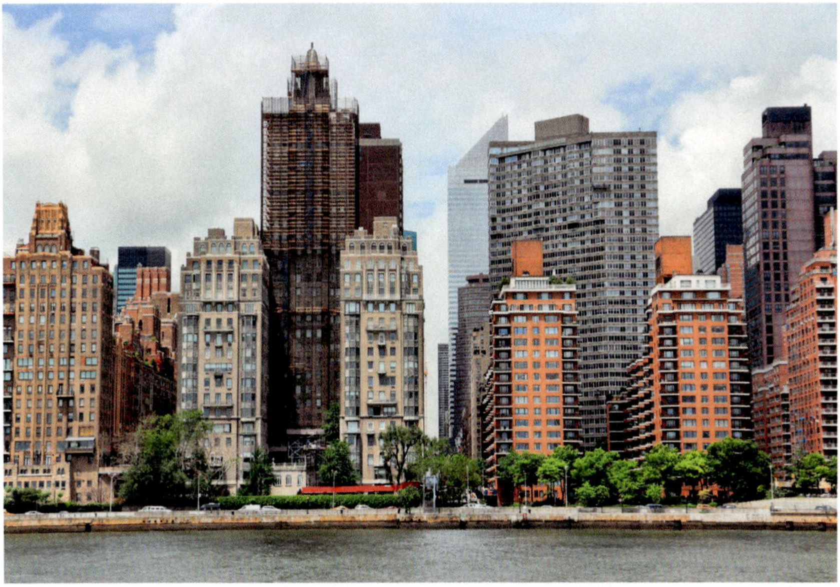

Adobe Photo

View of Sutton Place from the East River

New York City, envy of the civilized world, America's singular claim to the notion of an urban ideal, is not a city at all. It is a patchwork of a place—beauty, elegance, culture, the products of unrestricted urges of human creativity, stitched carefully together with poverty, mendacity, selfishness, and evil culled from the cast-off scraps of the efforts of people from everywhere to make a place for themselves. It is beautiful. I think the stitching is the key. With the common thread of mankind's need to belong, generations of seekers have meticulously sewn the pieces together into a sturdy patchwork whole with an allure that pulls at the human spirit.

Arlene and I fell under the spell of *The City* during multiple visits there for professional responsibilities related mostly to The American Thoracic Society. The process was gradual. New York does not seize your sensibilities suddenly. It is rarely love at first site. The place is too big for that. And too diverse. And business visits are too short and focused in time and space to venture very far beyond the margins proscribed by the people picking up the tab.

But even given those limitations, the allure filters through porous spots in your perimeter and draws you into the firmer substance of the place. We were victims of that process. Seduced by The City's penetrating reality, Arlene and I decided that we wanted to spend a lot of unencumbered time there and to do that we wanted to own a pied-à-terre in Manhattan, the epicenter of the place.

Zeitgeist, Janice and Manuel's gallery and office, graciously hosted a release party for one of my novels and during a lull in the proceedings, I mentioned to Manuel our interest in a NYC apartment. He disappeared for a few minutes and returned with the contact information for a Manhattan realtor who had sold a friend of the Zeitlins an apartment there and came highly recommended. A casual conversation with a friend set events in motion that we had not anticipated. We were still at the thinking stage, a ways yet, we thought, from the doing stage. But given our aging bodies and our recent downsizing from our Atlanta penthouse to more modest digs, the rationalization was easy enough.

Finding an apartment in a patchwork city on, at least by Manhattan standards, a limited budget, is no small task, even with expert professional help. Since Arlene and I were academic types, the Upper West Side came immediately to mind. I imagined a photograph of my rumpled self, backed by floor-to-ceiling bookcases stuffed to the gills with elite sounding titles, poring diligently over a stubborn computer. Serious sticker shock shattered that vision. And then there were the more adventurous patches—The Village, Soho. Same thing. Hard to compete with Taylor Swift and Meryl Streep on a couple of relatively paltry academic doctors' salaries.

The first Internet-derived spread of apartments that our realtor, Nicole Paikoff, showed us in her bulging notebook of flats that she thought we might like and even be able to afford, was a charming studio, nicely staged for sale, at the far end of Sutton Place South. We were completely unaware of the Sutton Place area but were struck with the atmospheric transition that occurred over the short block of Fifty-Fourth Street that ran east from a bustling First Avenue commercial district to dead end in the serene confines of an entirely residential area with wide sidewalks and idyllic riverside parks bathed in cool air wafting across the East River.

We later learned of the disparate array of notable figures who had lived at one time or another in the Sutton Place area—I.M. Pei, Bobby Short, Freddie Mercury, Marilyn Monroe and Arthur Miller, Aristotle Onassis, Mario Cuomo, Kurt Waldheim, among others. But they had been located mostly north of where we were looking, "the good part of Sutton Place as opposed to the Miami Beach looking part," Tom Wolfe calls it in a vignette from *Radical Chic and Mau-Mauing the Flak Catchers.*

Maybe more than a trifle starry-eyed from the possibility of realizing another dream, we bought the place that day to, I am sure, the surprise of both our realtor and the seller. Well, not really that day. It was after all a New York co-op, so there were the intricacies of co-op ownership to deal with—letters of reference, financial documents, meetings with the board, etc. We eventually cleared those hurdles and became the proud owners of a fantasy that had haunted us for several years.

We could not have picked a better place. I would never have expected to discover an oasis stitched into the fabric of a city that was constantly straining at the seams binding together its myriad elements. But Sutton Place was just that. Maybe it was the river? The residual footprints of the multi-gifted? The proximity to the patchwork of sublime and ridiculous?

Or maybe it was the irrepressible magic of our race that sometimes bursts forth as a gift from a friend who was expert at seeing all kinds of possibilities. Thanks, Manuel.

Opportunity

An Accidental Friend

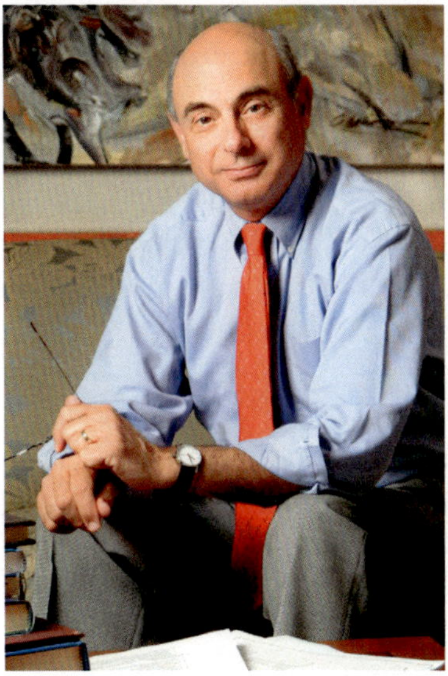

Jack Kearse/Emory University

Michael M.E. Johns

Bearing the indelible imprint of the Johns Hopkins ethos, I had long since gathered up my obligations and headed elsewhere when Mike Johns arrived in Baltimore to begin his illustrious career there. I imagine that we may have passed like ships in the night somewhere along our separate ways, but if so, neither of us noticed. We first met in Atlanta almost half a century after I took my leave of Baltimore.

He might have been a priest. A good Catholic boy from Detroit with an abiding desire to do something useful with his life, but without unlimited resources, might well have gone that route. And Mike had a go at the seminary. But it didn't take. I suspect that the prospect of lifelong celibacy wasn't a very powerful drawing card; there may have been other things that bothered him as well. For whatever reasons, upon facing a seminal divergence of the road to the priesthood and the road to something else, Mike chose something else. That road led him into medicine where he reckoned he could use his considerable talents while satisfying his need to improve the lots of his fellow humans and make a decent living in the process—do well by doing good. Even in his youth, Mike was a sharp cookie.

Why Atlanta after all those years? For almost three decades, I was on the faculty at Vanderbilt. I thought I would finish out my career there but wound up at Emory for the last ten years of my academic life as a result of the unpredictable vagaries of the academy. The people running the academic show inevitably change and bring with them different loyalties, interests, and personal attitudes that can reconfigure a place. Nearing the end of my long career as something of a star performer at what I considered my home institution, I fell victim to a new administration which was not so enamored of my efforts and probably of me as a person. It was no longer a place where I belonged. Wayne Alexander, chair of the Department of Medicine at Emory, offered me a job as vice chair for research, as well as a tenured position for Arlene, and we leapt at the chance to take on a new challenge in a new place.

Meanwhile, Mike had worked his way through the institutions of higher learning in his home state, emerging as an accomplished head and neck cancer surgeon, and moved on to Charlottesville where he distinguished himself and burnished his national reputation. As a result, he was eventually recruited to Hopkins in an effort to bring new energy to their flagging ear, nose and throat (ENT) department. He did that and, in the process, discovered an exceptional talent for organizing and managing a busy medical practice. Carefully observing how his department's faculty went about its business, he realized that patients were staying in the hospital much longer than necessary for some procedures and set about to establish the first Hopkins outpatient surgery program. The program saved money and made everybody happier. Such things do not go unnoticed by the impresarios of the medicine show, so in due time, Mike was appointed dean of the Johns Hopkins School of Medicine.

One does not wear such an august title lightly, and I don't think Mike was inclined to hide his talents anyway. Even had he been so inclined, it is unlikely that he would have been overlooked by other institutions who constantly trolled the marketplace for leaders who had proven themselves in demanding roles to be creative and successful. Mike was refined in the white-hot flame of academic politics at a top echelon institution while planting his footprints deep in the complexities of how the place functioned. When the folks at Emory entered the market for an executive vice president for health affairs, Mike Johns was not just a safe bet, he also promised to bring a new level of energy and imagination to a university that had sometimes been too comfortable reclining on its enormous Coca Cola-fed endowment.

Why would Mike pull up stakes, leave one of the most prestigious positions in American medicine, and head south, a long way from either Detroit or Baltimore, toward what must have seemed unfamiliar territory with new and unfamiliar challenges? This job was the alpha dog for the medical center, all right, but it was also, among other things, the top dog for the Schools of Public Health and Nursing and the head of the largest clinical program in Georgia. Why would he take on what sounded to any sane person like an impossible job? What was he thinking?

Fact is, he was probably salivating at the prospects. Mike thrived on challenge. Challenge was grist for his daunting energy mill. He took the job because he knew he could do it and was probably pretty sure that he could do it better than most. By the time I arrived in Atlanta, Mike was deeply ensconced in the place, already leaving his mark. My job was in the Department of Medicine, several administrative echelons below the rarefied atmosphere respired in the offices of the alpha dog. It took a while for our paths to cross. I think it was AIDS that, quite by accident, staged that unlikely encounter.

Even having spent most of my life involved in the process of scientific discovery, I'm still not sure exactly how major advances in medicine happen. How do the relative roles of knowledge and serendipity play into the often complex and obscure sequence of events that birth the eventual epiphany, the AHA! moment, when the scales fall from the scientists' eyes and they see clearly what their science has wrought. That must have happened at some point to Ray Schinazi and Dennis Liotta, Emory colleagues who discovered the antiviral drug that became the preferred lifelong treatment for HIV/AIDS. They must have been exhilarated at the prospect of rescuing so many from an ugly and certain death, but they were probably blissfully unaware of more peripheral potential of their discovery. The university sold the rights to the drug to Gilead Sciences, Inc., for an incomprehensible amount of money and with the proceeds, launched an institution-wide evaluation of what the university was about and what it could become. The theme for the medical center was *Predictive Health* and for reasons that I still don't know (I doubted that he even knew who I was at the time), Mike asked me to chair that part of the assessment.

So there was the AIDS drug that caused our professional paths to intersect, but I think the discovery of a shared affection for single malt Scotch whisky may have greased the skids toward friendship. At one of our weekly meetings meant to discuss progress with the Predictive Health initiative up there in the thin air of the top dog's suite of offices, the conversation drifted for unfathomable reasons to the topic of spirits distilled in the highlands of Scotland. Delighted to discover that the man running the whole medical enterprise was a card-carrying member of the brotherhood of lovers of Scotch whisky, I brought Mike a bottle of my favorite as a gift to our next meeting. There was a back story to my chosen favorite.

It would soon be dark in the small village on the isle of Islay, Queen of the Hebrides, off the north coast of Scotland. The shadows cast by the ruined castle sitting obstinately for centuries by the water were growing long and the sea, exhausted from its day-long assault on the grassy shore, murmured quietly of the coming night and the promise of tomorrow. The only commercial establishment in the village was a general store that seemed to sell everything one might need in such a place. It was also where anyone interested could pick up the key to the old castle with no collateral, only a promise to return it promptly. I guess people interested in the ruins of old castles tend to keep their word.

"A bottle of Laphroaig," I requested of the bearded store proprietor.

He smiled broadly and replied. "Bah, Laphraoig. We send all that stuff to America. Try a real whisky."

He retrieved a dark green bottle from a shelf behind where he stood and sat it with a resounding thud on the counter.

"Bunnahabhain!" he exclaimed. "Best damn Islay single malt you're apt to find."

Of the boundless array of choices, I wondered how he made such a decisive claim. What was so special about this particular bottle? Was the invading American tourist being challenged to choose a more authentic favorite? Why? The rotund green bottle was attractive, but what about the nuances of color, texture, peatiness, etc.? How about a wee dram to convince me, laddie? In the end, as with many of life's choices, it was the story that mattered most. I was sold on Bunnahabhain Scotch even before popping the cork and inhaling that distinctive sharp peaty aroma characteristic of the Islay malts. Had to be the magic of the story.

So, at my next meeting with Mike, I delivered the bottle of my favorite libation. That probably helped launch a friendship and a collaboration that is still vibrant. We worked hard on the Predictive Health initiative until our retirement. We co-authored two books (*Predictive Health*, Basic Books, and *The Good Doctor*, Seven Stories Press). We have spent many sunny afternoons sipping Scotch from Mike's impressive collection on the terrace of his beautiful Brookhaven home while ruminating on the current situation in American medicine and in the world at large. Although the pandemic and other things have kept us physically apart for a while now, we stay in touch. I suspect we always will. Real friendships endure.

Predictive Health

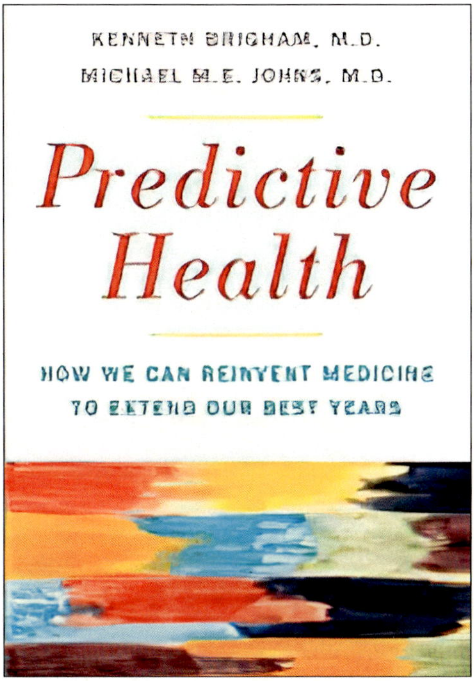

2012 book by Drs. Brigham and Johns

By forcing health care to function in a marketplace driven by a reward system that ignores the value of doing good for its own sake, we have squandered the potential of scientific excellence, advanced technology, and enormous investments of valuable resources by our choice of metrics to evaluate what we are doing. Health care does not play by the usual economic rules. Simple concepts of supply and demand do not work to the good of society when applied to something that does not fit into a product box and is a universal human right. Faced with the health care challenge, the vaunted marketplace as the principal determinant of how things work crumbles before our eyes, the shards scattering to the four winds to be exploited for gain by a fragmented and myopic pseudo-system that serves its people poorly and costs too much. Other civilized countries have figured this out and have done something about it. Why have we Americans been so slow to realize what we are doing? Why don't we care enough to be about fixing it?

Although I still don't know the answers to those questions, nor to the larger question of how do you fix it even if we had the social will to do so, a couple of years after my arrival in Atlanta, I was given the chance to converse about the problem with a broad swath of experts from across Emory University as part of the most encompassing and intense effort to define a future course for an institution that I had ever had the privilege of participating in. It was an interesting glimpse into how university faculties with diverse expertise, personalities, interests, ambitions, and *modi operandi* behave when drawn outside their usual comfort zone and asked to talk seriously about things beyond their ken. They didn't always distinguish themselves.

The idea was to articulate a few transcendent themes and then engage the entire spectrum of university disciplines in prolonged discussions of the nature, definition, and academic implications of each theme with careful attention to how multidisciplinarity could identify and enhance novel actions that emerged from the discussions. The medicine-related theme was *Predictive Health and Society*.

I suppose that for anyone familiar with such activities in the business world, the process would have been predictable. Battalions of expensive consultants invaded the campus for a couple of months. They arrived bearing their neat packets of multicolored magic markers, big paper tablets mounted on easels, red rubber balls in their pockets for tossing at drowsy members of their audience to get their attention, and what sounded like a tightly scripted patter that might have functioned in some settings but that often seemed to me ill-suited to an academic institution and having little relevance to a productive discussion of the future of medicine in America. My role in this whole thing was to lead the discussions on the Predictive Health theme (which were actually led for the most part by the visiting consultants), and to produce a document that summarized the process and the conclusions that would serve to inform whoever was going to decide about how to advance the academic goals of the university.

I tried to do that and we made progress, I think, mostly despite the consultants. Although I was named director of the project, it was a special interest of Mike Johns, Emory's executive vice president for health affairs, top dog on the medicine side of things. His support for it opened doors that otherwise would have been barricaded shut by provincial and personal interests and faculty politics. For example, Don Giddens, dean of the School of Engineering at Georgia Tech, volunteered to commit faculty and other resources to a Predictive Health Institute that would be a joint effort of the two institutions. Mike coaxed a million dollars from a local family foundation that was added to the three million allotted to this theme by the university, so we had some resources to start to test whether Predictive Health as we had defined it was as powerful a concept as we thought.

For a while, it looked like we might be onto something. The Emory-Georgia Tech Center for Health Discovery and Well-Being (CHDWB) was established as a project that would serve as a proof of principle that defining human health as a positive condition, something other than the absence of disease, and measuring some of the defining variables over time would identify early deviations from health that predicted when something worse was in the offing that could be nipped in the bud—more health, less cost. It worked, at least for a while. More than five hundred essentially healthy people were followed with annual measurements of a variety of health-related variables over several years. The data were analyzed and reported by scores of faculty from more than a dozen disciplines. Although predictive algorithms were not simple and information we thought would be informative sometimes wasn't, it was a start.

Enter the unpredictability of the academic enterprise. Predictive Health champion Mike Johns became chancellor of Emory University and was replaced as the executive vice president for health affairs by an executive who had other priorities. There was a major turnover in leadership at Georgia Tech that ended in Dean Giddens retiring from the engineering school and taking with him any hope that the envisioned commitments from that institution would happen. Although some fragment of the CHDWB continues and the valuable database still exists as an investigative resource, the original vision of a grand new approach to health and well-being that energized some of us at the time is now a pale institutional memory.

Not that the basic idea is dead. It has in fact, under various guises—personalized medicine, precision medicine, e.g.—become a dominant concept among future oriented university medical centers and in the halls of government agencies that direct health care research and policy. The Atlanta universities were there before it was a popular place to be, poised on the penetrating point of the cutting edge and needing only the deliberate thrust of conviction by confident leaders to set in motion a change for the better in the health care world.

The plague of missed opportunity still haunts those of us who were players in that scene. I fear that we bear some of the burden of our country's excruciatingly ponderous consideration of its citizens' health and well-being. Our failure to follow through on the deal when we had the chance may have given the naysayers another excuse to procrastinate. A contract between our government and the people to whom it is obligated that guarantees the human right of health care to every citizen is inevitable; common sense and morality demand it and the politics will eventually come around. We might have missed a chance to hurry that process along.

The elaborate Emory University self-evaluation produced a nicely articulated mission statement that is short enough to be appealing although I'm not sure there is anything unique about the content. But I can't see much change yet in how we go about caring for the health and well-being of anyone. Too bad.

Non Finito

Cancer Redux

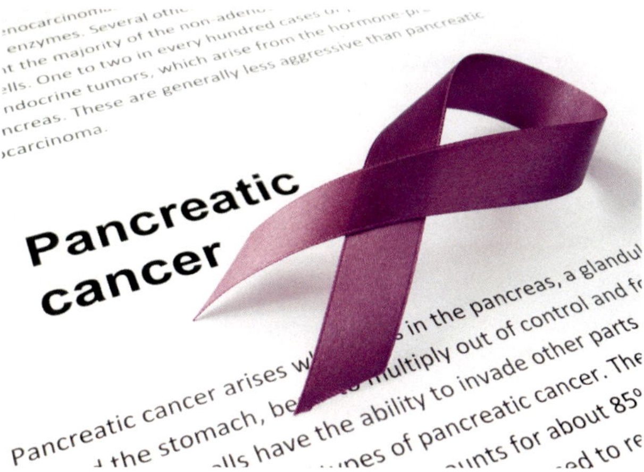

AdVitalii Vodolazskyi/Adobe Photo

Life is not a long and winding road.
The road is short and as straight as a poison arrow.
Abner [Hal Holbrook's aging character in That Evening Sun (2009)].

Not that I'm complaining. I've had a full and long life. But as an observer of the human condition, it seems to me that one potentially fatal cancer per lifetime is more than enough to round out the experience of living. It only takes a single, serious cheek by jowl encounter with the Grim Reaper to focus one's undivided attention on the things that matter and to fully engage the essence of one's humanity in the business of living or dying, depending on how the story turns out. If you make it through number one, isn't a second closeup encounter with malignancy, a round two, a waste of the remaining potential of a life that has already learned most of the lessons in cancer's pedagogic portfolio? Why do I need to repeat a course that I've taken before and aced?

Why, after all these years, the angel on my shoulder, sounding more than a little exasperated, whispers softly into my good ear, *do you still insist on trying to make sense of all this? Forget it. Things happen because they are in the neighborhood of your lifepath at the time you're passing by, and if you imagine them into a logical pattern that looks familiar, you will manufacture nonsense.*

"I know, I know," I thought while secretly wishing that the angel on my shoulder had more palatable advice to offer. The rascal was starting to sound like she was enjoying this. Maybe I needed a little nonsense those days.

Arlene arranged a celebration of my eightieth birthday at our studio in Venice with the people whom I love most in the world. We rented an extra apartment in the same palazzo where our flat was located, and Heather and her husband, Josh, and Arlene's brother and his wife (Richard and Lorna) joined us there. Our Venice friend, Sarah Sherwood, arranged several outings and we located two local women who came to the apartment and cooked a wonderfully creative and very Italian birthday dinner for the group. There was lots of bonding time in a setting that nurtures such things. I had some special time with Heather and came to appreciate Josh even more if that was possible. I could not have imagined a more memorable birthday. *To love and be loved.* I kept thinking of Arlene's understanding of our purpose for being. I couldn't think of a better one.

But the world kept turning, a cosmic fact that takes on additional meaning as the rotations accumulate and their consequences accrete. Near the end of our stay in Italy, I began to feel ill and to lose weight. By the time we arrived back in Atlanta, Arlene observed that I was jaundiced. Jaundice in an eighty-year-old man does not bode well. The diagnosis was quickly established by the immediate attention of my long-time internist, David Roberts, and the surgeon whom he favored, David Kooby,—adenocarcinoma of the pancreas, a disease that is *not cured but managed,* according to Walid Shaib, the oncologist to whom I was referred.

I was not encouraged by the prospects. How does one manage a fatal disease? I couldn't think of a management strategy with an outcome that I was ready to accept. It sounded to me like my doctors were just going to do what they could to ease my path to the inevitable after the management approach had run its course. I thought that was ceding too much control of the outcome to the cancer. Turning over one's future to malignancy was likely, it seemed to me, to guarantee a malignant future. Let's not throw up our hands just yet, guys.

Arlene was as distraught as I was by the situation, but she was determined to keep a positive mindset and was equally determined to do everything she could to see that I did the same. After all, we were in this thing together and she was ready to take on whatever challenges we faced with the full force of her being. That had worked before. But it had been a while. I wasn't sure how many *get out of mortality free cards* Arlene had stashed away, but if she was confident that her supply was not yet exhausted, who was I to question it?

There is a chance for a surgical cure of this disease if the cancer is in the head of the pancreas, the part at the east end of the organ (toward the host's right side). A cancer in the tail (on the west side) may require removing all of the organ which eliminates some vital functions like the proper metabolism of sugars and processing fats so that they move through the gut and on to wherever they're supposed to wind up. You just can't do some important things without at least a sizeable fraction of a normal pancreas.

However, if the tumor is in the head of the organ, it is possible to cut it out along with a part of the pancreas, a big chunk of the neighboring intestine, and some other stuff, reassemble everything, and leave most things working well enough to avoid diabetes, bad fat absorption, etc. This is called a pancreatico-duodenectomy or a Whipple procedure (named after the surgeon who invented it). I can assure you that such a procedure is not for the timid of constitution. The short-term consequences are agonizing and in the longer run, all those rearrangements of your insides change your life forever.

That's the situation under normal circumstances. But when I was the operatee, circumstances were anything but normal. On March 16, 2020, all Emory hospitals went on full shutdown due to the coronavirus pandemic, which was rapidly taking over the lion's share of the medical care facilities in Atlanta and elsewhere, requiring draconian procedural changes to minimize viral spread. Full shutdown meant deferral of all elective surgeries (including many cancer surgeries) and exclusion of all nonpatients except health care personnel from the hospitals. No visitors. No exceptions. About that time, I had finished my pre-operative chemotherapy and tolerated it well. Arlene and I were psyching ourselves up for dealing with major surgery, probably my only chance at a cure.

Compliments of the thriving coronavirus, the surgery was delayed while continuing chemotherapy. Finally, early in the morning of May 15, Arlene dropped me off reluctantly at the front door of Emory St. Joseph's Hospital. We parted with a very wet embrace and separated our ways for what turned out to be more than a month of surgery and stormy recovery for me and the pain of separation and anxiety about the unknown for her. Heather and Josh would have dropped everything and come to Atlanta but for the travel restrictions imposed by the virus, so their support had to be limited to the telephone. Mike Johns was a reliable and rock-solid support for Arlene. But the collusion of the cancer and the virus that ripped us mercilessly from each other's arms and forced us to our own devices to handle the most serious and threatening event in our otherwise idyllic relationship, was as close to devastation as I cared to experience.

During that long month in the hospital, much of it spent in pain and disorientation, there were times when I would have questioned whether it was all worth it had it not been for Arlene's constant reassuring voice on the phone. She stayed in touch with Heather and relayed messages of intense concern and support from her and Josh. I had excellent medical and surgical care essential to my recovery, but I am convinced that love was the source of strength and endurance that made the crucial difference, that saved my life. But for the grace of those I *love and am loved by* my endgame would have come essentially alone in a sterile hospital room lost amid the babble and clatter of a failed emergency code—a route to the other side that I would strongly advise avoiding if possible. You don't want to do that dance if there's any way around it.

Despite all the drama, here I am now well over a year after being told I had pancreatic cancer and feeling quite well, thank you. The COVID-19 behavioral restrictions have done me the favor of having Arlene working from home most of the time, here for me when I need her, which is pretty much always. The same virus has kept us from the pleasure of sharing personal time with family and close friends and from our getaway studios in New York and Venice. But it has given me time to settle into our Atlanta home and to recover almost back to my old self. Chemotherapy continues for a while, but I still tolerate it well. And I am writing again.

So even though I aced the Grim Reaper's course on the first go-round, maybe I had more to learn. A deeper lesson that you can learn only when the road gets "short and as straight as a poison arrow": *There is a time to call in some of your chits from those who love you and to start doling out to those you love whatever you have left to give.*

To the angel on my shoulder: Okay, I made it through the Grim Reaper's second shot (at least so far, so good) and maybe learned something. But don't get the idea that I need a third one.

Non Finito!

Answers

Afterlife

Well, not quite there yet (still *Non Finito*, some winding up to do), but according to the rules that human biology generally plays by, it can't be all that long. So it's timely, I think, now that the road is short and straight, to reflect on the last eighty-odd years, to mine them for any pithy observations about the course of human existence that might be at least interesting and perhaps even useful to you fellow travelers, trudging along in lockstep with Father Time somewhere on the path that is headed in that direction. You will get there. We all will. It's just a matter of time until time doesn't matter.

Apart from whatever wisdom comes with the passage of time and experience, I have no particular qualifications for reaching conclusions about human existence. But I'm not sure anyone else does either, so that I figure that I'm about as qualified as the next old fellow. Anyway, for what they're worth, here are some thoughts born of reflections on an accidental life.

There is no certain answer to why. "For now we see through a glass, darkly..." The apostle Paul uses the metaphor to contrast faith and knowledge for the Christians at Corinth. We mortals can't know for certain the answers to a lot of *whys*, the reasons for many events that determine who we are and how we live. Why was I born in a particular place to particular parents? Why did I happen to be black or white or brown or yellow? Why am I the product of a close-knit, loving family that nurtured me to a productive adulthood instead of being born into a dysfunctional family that abandoned me in my youth, leaving me to my own devices to survive the mean streets of life? Why do I believe in a God ... or not? If there are rational (or irrational) explanations for major determinants of who we are and what we do, I think a lot of them are beyond the ken of us mortal beasts.

We can't *know*, but we can *believe*. Probably most of the eight billion of us choose to believe something about the meaning and purpose of our earthly existence. There are many options, although where and under whose care and influence we have been forced to confront the world no doubt limit the possibilities. But you may find comfort in choosing one of the countless proposed answers to *why* as an eternal truth that guides your life. If so, and that brings you peace and happiness with your fellow humans in the real world, you deserve congratulations and the support of others. Of course, you owe it to your brothers and sisters to respond to them with the same acceptance and concern that you expect, even if they have chosen other spiritual paths or have arrived at altogether different conclusions about the meaning of life. There is no credible way for any of us to claim exclusivity for our chosen view. Perhaps there are many truths. Who knows?

The answer to why not is why not. Before you get too annoyed, let me explain what I mean by the tautology. If there is no knowable *why*, then the universal answer to the questioning mind must be *why not*. What is *is*. We live in a real world and must accept reality if we are to find any equanimity there. Could things have happened some other way? Probably. Reality may be fickle on occasion. But things didn't happen some other way. They happened as they did and getting too troubled by that, too fixated on other possibilities, is not likely to make you more comfortable with your humanity.

Why me? ... Why not! When, for hyperbolic example, the forces that be shift the earth's tectonic plates in ways that open vast crevasses that swallow innocent people, vaporizing them in the planet's fiery bowels, why would someone you love be one of the victims? Well, things like that sometimes happen and you have to deal with them as best you can. If you are looking for personal guilt or, maybe worse, some conscious diabolical force that punishes innocence and the love of humans for each other, you will find them only in your imagination. There is no reason to feel personal guilt (earthquakes and even lesser misfortunes are usually not your fault). And as for your imagined diabolical force, you'd be better off forgetting about any such thing and engaging that fertile imagination in something more constructive and more connected to what is. Grieve your loss and live the life that reality grants you. You can count on reality … for as long as it lasts anyway.

"***Pay attention***, Dad," a tenish-year-old Heather once instructed her distracted father.

Good advice with much broader implications than my young daughter probably realized at the time. *You can see a lot just by looking* is Yogi Berra's folksier take on the same subject. The point is that fully engaging your five senses with the world where you live will bring beauty and awe into your life and will smooth the edges of the harsher realities that will inevitably come your way. Satchmo declares "What a Wonderful World." Who wants to argue with Satchmo?

Take a side trip. You have limited say about the course and circumstances of your Big Trip, the trek in step with Father Time toward whatever, but you can escape the old guy's clutches for a bit on occasion (he will hold your place in line) and explore the territory beyond. Do it. Take a side trip once in a while. And take it seriously. Saturate your senses with what is. See, hear, feel, taste, smell the realities of our spectacular planet and your fellow humans who live with you there. You'll be surprised at how much beauty and good you were at risk of missing when you spent so much of your feverishly evaporating time pondering unknowables. Right on, Satchmo!

Be kind. I confirm this admonition from the late Welsh writer Jan Morris. Her *free dance* through an extraordinary life was much more imaginative than mine, but I think we wound up at similar places. We both learned that the importance of kindness, to yourself and others, looms large as the road gets short.

Love and be loved. Whatever answers you choose to believe to life's existential questions, here, I think, is the essential meaning of humanity, the reason we exist. It makes sense of what otherwise can be chaos, nonsense, and bafflement: *To experience the ecstatic reality of loving another human being and the transcendent peace of being loved without condition or purpose.* If you can master this part of living well, the rest of it may not matter very much.